EMMA

PLANT BASED COOKBOOK FOR BEGINNERS

123 Easy Recipes for Restore your Energy, Detox your Body and Lose Weight with Natural Ingredients.

No part of this book may be reproduced or transmitted in any form or by any means, electronic or mechanical, including photocopying, recording or by any information storage and retrieval system, without written permission from the author, except for the inclusion of brief quotations in a review.

Limit of Liability and Disclaimer of Warranty: The publisher has used its best efforts in preparing this book, and the information provided herein is provided "as is." This book is designed to provide information and motivation to our readers. It is sold with the understanding that the publisher is not engaged to render any type of psychological, legal, or any other kind of professional advice. The content of each article is the sole expression and opinion of its author, and not necessarily that of the publisher. No warranties or guarantees are expressed or implied by the publisher's choice to include any of the content in this volume. Neither the publisher nor the individual author(s) shall be liable for any physical, psychological, emotional, financial, or commercial damages, including, but not limited to, special, incidental, consequential or other damages. Our views and rights are the same: You are responsible for your own choices, actions, and results.

Copyright © 2020 by Emma Morales. All rights reserved.

Introduction

Chapter 1: What is Plant-Based Diet?

Chapter 2: How a Plant-Based Diet Can Detox Your Body and Restore Your Energy.

   Key principles of plant-based diet

Chapter 3: 5 Reasons To Follow A Plant-Based Diet For Weight Loss

Chapter 4: What to Eat and What To Avoid

   Foods to avoid

Chapter 5: Breakfast and Smoothies

   Green Breakfast Smoothie

   Blueberry Lemonade Smoothie

   Berry Protein Smoothie

   Blueberry and Chia Smoothie

   Lettuce Mix Green Shake

   Basil and Pine Nuts Shake

   Rosemary-Lemon Garden Greens Smoothie

   Lemon-Cilantro Greens Shake

   Blackberry-Chocolate Shake

   Strawberry-Coconut Shake

   Berry Overload Shake

Mediterranean Breakfast Burrito

Homemade Granola

Breakfast Quinoa with Figs and Honey

Maple Walnut Teff Porridge

Chapter 6: Main Dishes

Black Bean Stuffed Sweet Potatoes

Black Bean and Quinoa Salad

Grilled Zucchini with Tomato Salsa

Eggplant Parmesan

Coconut Chickpea Curry

Mediterranean Chickpea Casserole

Sweet Potato and White Bean Skillet

Kung Pao Brussels Sprouts

Balsamic-Glazed Roasted Cauliflower

Stuffed Sweet Potato

Potatoes with Nacho Sauce

Veggie Kabobs

Summer Pesto Pasta

Linguine with Wild Mushrooms

Edamame and Noodle Salad

Pilaf with Garbanzos and Dried Apricots

Avocado and Lime Bean Bowl

Chapter 7: Soups and Stew

- Sweet Potato, Corn and Jalapeno Bisque
- Creamy Pea Soup with Olive Pesto
- Spinach Soup with Dill and Basil
- Coconut Watercress Soup
- Roasted Red Pepper and Butternut Squash Soup
- Tomato Pumpkin Soup
- Cauliflower Spinach Soup
- Avocado Mint Soup
- Creamy Squash Soup
- Zucchini Soup
- Creamy Celery Soup
- Avocado Cucumber Soup
- Garden Vegetable Stew
- Moroccan Vermicelli Vegetable Soup
- Moroccan Vegetable Stew
- Autumn Medley Stew
- Black Bean Soup with Sweet Potato

Chapter 8: Salads

- Cucumber Edamame Salad
- Best Broccoli Salad
- Rainbow Orzo Salad

Broccoli Pasta Salad

Eggplant & Roasted Tomato Farro Salad

Summer Corn Salad

Best Tomato and Avocado Salad

Sweet Pepper Panzanella

Purple Potato and Green Bean Salad

Spinach and Mashed Tofu Salad

Chapter 9: Side Dishes

Garden Patch Sandwiches on Multigrain Bread

Garden Salad Wraps

Marinated Mushroom Wraps

Tamari Toasted Almonds

Avocado and Tempeh Bacon Wraps

Stuffed Cherry Tomatoes

Spicy Black Bean Dip

French Onion Pastry Puffs

Salsa Fresca

Lemon and Garlic Marinated Mushrooms

Garlic Toast

Vietnamese-Style Lettuce Rolls

Chapter 10: Pasta and Noodles

Pasta with Roasted Red Pepper Sauce

Macaroni and Cheese

Veggies Soba Noodles with Marinated Tofu

Cambodian Vegetable Stir-Fry

Roasted Garlic Tomato Spaghetti with Garlic Parmesan Bread Crumbs

Zoodle Pad Thai

Peanut Vegetable Noodle Bowl

Garlic Pasta with Roasted Brussels Sprouts And Tomatoes

Veggies and Noodle Bowl with Mushrooms

Veggie Pasta

Summer Garlic Scape and Zucchini Pasta

Sun Dried Tomato Pesto Pasta

Zucchini Pasta with Spicy Tomato and Lentil Sauce

Lemon Pepper Asparagus Pasta

Butternut Squash Fettuccine

Collard Green Spaghetti

Pasta Salad with Tahini Dressing

Spicy Vegan Pasta with Sausage

Chapter 11: Vegetables

Tahini Broccoli Slaw

Steamed Cauliflower

Roasted Cauliflower Tacos

Cajun Sweet Potatoes

Creamy Mint-Lime Spaghetti Squash

Smoky Coleslaw

Simple Sesame Stir-Fry

Mediterranean Hummus Pizza

Baked Brussels Sprouts

Minted Peas

Spicy Fruit and Veggie Gazpacho

Maple Dijon Burgers

Caramelized Root Vegetables

Sushi-Style Quinoa

Pepper Medley

Sautéed Citrus Spinach

Chapter 12: Snacks/Desserts

Strawberry Mango Shave Ice

Chocolate Avocado Mousse

Fudge

Chocolate Chip Cookies

Pumpkin Ice Cream

Sautéed Pears

Raw Vegan Chocolate Fruit Balls

- Baked Sesame Fries
- No-Bake Coconut Chia Macaroons
- Avocado Lassi
- Vegan Fudge Revel Bars

Chapter 13: Energizing Drinks

- Gingerbread Latte
- Black Forest Shake
- Lemon Ginger Detox Tea
- Carrot Pineapple Ginger Juice
- Strawberry Shrub Mocktail
- Strawberry Margaritas
- Fresh Mint Julep

Conclusion

Introduction

The problem faced by many isn't about finding the desire to diet with whole-plant foods, but how to break the addiction to heavily focused meaty foods. In this book, i guide you in the simplest ways to transition from regular eating into this new and healthier space.

The goal is to find the perfect replacement for animal products and make your options countless.

In this book, i disconnect unexciting eating practices from dieting but create recipes that follow the trends of regular diet while incorporating plant-based foods into them. Shouldn't dieting be a fun adventure? I will ensure that the recipes make you tick! Their aromas are incredible, they taste heavenly, and yet communicate a state of wellness from your tongue down through your guts. And they are satisfying!

Still not sure if you can commit to eating plant-based foods100 percent? No need to worry. The following chapters will show you in detail how you do not need to approach a plant-based diet with an all-or-nothing attitude. Rest assured that every step you take is a step closer to lowered risks of developing chronic diseases, and higher energy levels through a plant-based diet that you can stick with for the rest of your longer and healthier life.

No other way gives me more pleasure than to share these recipes with you. It is my desire and a promise that you will feel transformed physically, mentally, emotionally, and spiritually as you diet this fun way. I ensured that each ingredient used for the recipes is easily accessible at your local grocery store. The cooking processes are also seamless and cook in the quickest time possible. I am enthusiastic about the positive impact of this cookbook on your life and looking forward to all the good stuff that you are yet to experience.

So, why hesitate further? Start cooking now and journey think of a world without meats and processed foods, how will you work around them?

Chapter 1: What is Plant-Based Diet?

The question is more like this: what is the difference between plant-based diet and veganism?

Both food approaches do not involve meat consumption. But if vegans are ethically motivated, those who follow a plant-based diet also reject everything that is processed on an industrial and unhealthy level.

However, a plant-based diet is based on the consumption of fruit, vegetables, and whole grains and avoiding (or minimizing) the intake of animal products and processed foods. This means that even vegan desserts made with refined sugar or bleached flour are not included in a plant-based diet. In short, both diets avoid eating hamburgers (the kind with meat or chicken patties), but for different reasons: vegans because they do not eat meat and those who follow a plant-based diet because they do not eat processed foods and hydrogenated fats and do so for health reasons.

While there is no doubt that humans were meant to be eating fruits, vegetables and nuts from the beginning, a shift took place that introduced a large confusion, mixing humans with the omnivore species.

Scientifically speaking, a plant-based diet is much more beneficial and less harmful for humans, which is why it is recommended to shift from meat to whole grains, legumes, vegetables and other nutritional foods of this kind.

Switching to a plant-based diet is beneficial for many reasons. If you are suffering from any kind of illnesses or have obesity issues, you should focus on a plant-based diet as a way to better your health and reduce your symptoms, if not cure the illness completely. Nutrition is a powerful tool that can be used for great purposes, such as helping relieve pain and health problems, improving metabolism and the immune system, as well as strengthen your body and improve your mood.

Even if you do not have any health-related problems, you should transition to a plant-based diet as a means of preventive health building. The natural ingredients such as fruits, legumes or vegetables are full of nutritional values needed for the everyday functioning of our systems. In all cases, whole food is always better than processed food, as it does not contain any chemicals or unnatural substances that could be harmful to our health.

Besides boosting your health, a plant-based diet can decrease the risks of many diseases, among them the most serious ones such as heart diseases, type 2 diabetes and certain types of cancers.

Many studies at research facilities have proven these statements to be correct, such as, for example, a study conducted in Jama internal medicine, which tracked over 70 000 people and their eating habits. This study has proven that a plant-based diet can significantly improve your health and lengthen your life as well. Therefore, switching to a plant-based diet is one of the best things you can do for yourself and your overall well-being.

People who consume plant-based products have a lower risk of developing diseases or having strokes because of the fiber, vitamins and minerals that come along with a plant-based diet. The fiber, vitamins and minerals, as well as healthy fats, are essential substances your body needs in order to function properly. Plant-based diet thus improve the blood lipid levels and better your brain health as well. There is a significant decrease in bad cholesterol in people who follow a plant-based diet.

It is never too late to change your diet! Whether you are 18, 36 or 50, it is still recommended to switch to a plant-based diet, as it is never too late to do so! These diets have quick and effective results that you will be noticing even after the first week of eating only plant-based meals.

The first results you will notice will be the sense of accomplishment and satisfaction that comes with following a healthy diet.

You will notice your mood has improved, in addition to not feel heavy after a meal, but instead feeling full and satisfied and yet energetic. After a period of following a plant-based diet, you will begin to notice the health benefits of doing so. Your health-related problems will be reduced and you will feel a significant relief in terms of pains or discomfort you have been having.

What is important to know when switching to a plant-based diet is that you are not going to be on any kind of deprivation diet. Many people relate plant-based diet as a diet where you are depriving yourself of meat and dairy. However, when you switch to a plant-based diet you will not feel like you are missing anything, since your taste will adapt to your new eating habits. This will lead to you finding foods delicious that you maybe even disliked before. The human body is adapting constantly to the different inputs, and after a while, plant-based food will feel tasty and natural to you. The foods prepared of the healthy, nutritional ingredients are very delicious, especially if you follow the right recipes. Stick through this diet guide to learn some great plant-based diet recipes you can include in your transition program. Once you see the benefits of the plant-based diet and try some of the specialties, you will never want to go back to your eating habits again.

Transitioning from a meat to a plant-based diet is not as difficult as everyone thinks. You can do it gradually, by increasing your fruit and vegetable intake while decreasing your meat and dairy intake. Minimizing meat consumption at first will make the transition seem effortless later, as you don't have to introduce drastic changes immediately.

Therefore, your diet will be based on fruits, vegetables, tubers, whole grains and legumes. You can start implementing these changes by replacing meat in your favorite recipes and dishes with mushrooms or beans. Gradually, you will completely lose the habit of consuming meat and switch to a full plant-based diet. To help your transition process, you should add more calories of legumes, whole grains and vegetables to your everyday routine, as that will make you feel full and thus reduce your desire to eat meat and dairy.

As soon as you start switching your diet you will notice how positively your body reacts to receiving all the nutrients it needs to function properly. The foods you should be focusing on include beans, that is, all legumes, berries, broccoli, cabbage, collards, nuts and kale.

Before we get into the detailed, 4-week program for switching to a plant-based diet, here are a few tips that will help you make the transition easily.

Include fruits and vegetables in every meal of the day. Instead of snacking on chocolate bars, switch to fruit or nutritional bars. Remember, an apple a day keeps the doctor away!

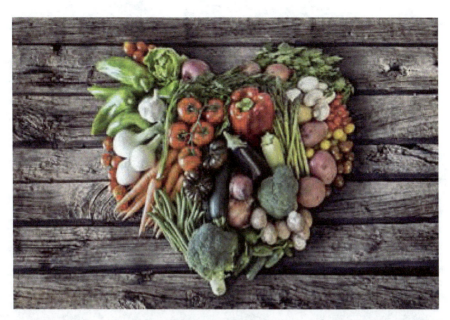

Downsize your meat servings gradually. Put less meat on your plate and more veggies. Make sure that the ¾ of the plate consists of plant-based ingredients!

You can slowly transition by introducing two or three meat-free days to your week plan. As time goes by you will get used to this system and you will be able to skip meat more often, until fully switching to the plant-based diet.

In addition to the many medical benefits of switching to a plant-based diet, there are also some truly powerful and indisputable cosmetic benefits as well.

Many studies have shown that there is a significant and strong link between the consumption of dairy products like milk, butter, or cheese, and undesirable skin conditions like acne, eczema, and early signs of aging.

Milk contains many similar properties to the hormone testosterone due to other hormones like progesterone making their way into the milk. It is thought that these hormones stimulate the oil glands of the skin, especially the face. An excess of sebum, or oil, is produced and thus acne occurs. This excess oil clogs your pores and can lead to other troublesome skin blemishes such as blackheads and whiteheads. This continuous cycle of clogged pores, blemishes, and acne takes a lot out of your skin and can cause scarring and stress. This can lead to signs of premature aging and skin loses its elasticity and vitality. Many people who switch to a plant-based diet notice an incredibly rapid improvement in the condition of their skin. People who have suffered from acne and started eating plant-based foods have noticed their skin clear significantly. This is in no way by chance. Cutting out or greatly reducing dairy can really help give your skin a new lease on life. If you are struggling with acne and have tried nearly everything under the sun such as harsh chemicals, expensive facials and skin treatments, or countless different brands claiming to heal your skin problems, something as simple as a plant-based diet may be the answer you've been searching for.

Followers of a plant-based diet have also raved about the excellent anti-aging benefits of the diet. Collagen, something our bodies naturally produce in abundance when we are young, is the key factor of what makes skin supple, resilient, firm, and have elasticity. As we get older, collagen production slows and our skin suffers as a result, becoming prone to sagginess and thinness. While this is a natural and inevitable part of life, collagen loss does not have to be so drastic as we age. A plant-based diet has been proven to boost collagen in your body by providing all of the important nutrients and amino acids that make up collagen and how it is produced. In a sense, subscribing to a plant-based diet is kind of like taking a dip in the fountain of youth! Fruits and vegetables like kale, broccoli, asparagus, spinach, grapefruit, lemons, and oranges are chock-full of vitamin c which is an extremely important component in producing the amino acids that make up collagen. The kind of lean protein found in nuts is important in keeping collagen around, adding to skin cell longevity and resilience. Red vegetables like tomatoes, beets, and red peppers all contain lycopene which is a kind of antioxidant that protects skin from the sun while simultaneously increases collagen production. Foods rich in zinc such as certain seeds and whole grains also promote collagen because the mineral repairs damaged cells and reduces inflammation. So many of the plant-based staples contain incredible amounts of all these collagen-boosting nutrients that you do not even have to go out of your way to seek them out. It is all right there in front of you! Looking and feeling younger has never been so easy. It really does start with the internal to make the external radiant and glowing, outer beauty starts from within.

In short, there are no two ways about it - switching to a plant-based diet is good for your heart, your health, your mind, and even your physical appearance! The facts of the matter are undeniable. Plant foods contain so many of the incredibly good nutrients that our bodies need to function properly. Making these foods a priority and centering your meals around them rather than just eating vegetables as an occasional side dish or a piece of fruit every now and then makes a huge difference in your health. By eating a diet heavy on meat, dairy, and other animal products and processed foods, it is easy to miss out on the wonderfully beneficial vitamins, minerals, antioxidants, and other nutrients that are in fruits, vegetables, legumes, tubers, grains, nuts, and seeds. Switching to a plant-based diet gives you the opportunity to obtain all of these healthful ingredients that will without a doubt lead you to a better, more fulfilling life.

Chapter 2: How a Plant-Based Diet Can Detox Your Body and Restore Your Energy.

It is essential to understand that a plant-based meal plan does not necessarily mean permanently eliminating animal products from your diet. It involves incorporating more and more plants and vegetables in your diet. It is a way of eating to satisfaction while not denying your body the essential nutrients it requires. Perception is in mind. Therefore, before one decides to stick to a plant-based meal, it is imperative to feed in your thinking that it is the best for your body, mind, and soul. That way, you'll start developing taste and liking for the plant-based meal, and with time, you will find it sweet and very fulfilling.

A plant-based meal has been used over the years both for therapeutic or just nutritional value. There are some vegetables which you may not find tasty, delicious, or sweet. The bitter plant adding fresh herb seasoning, and some can even be blended when making a smoothie. Always try to make it in a way that you can comfortably consume because sometimes it's not very sweet to the mouth but very good to the body.

If we eat a lot of plants, it means we are getting vitamins, fiber, and phytochemicals. These are nutrients that our bodies fall short of, thus keeping us away from taking a lot of supplements. While vegan meal emphasizes strictly eating plant-based food and zero animal product, plant-based meal incorporates animal protein but in minimal quantity. Plant-based meal thus is very accommodative and less restricting thus creates smooth and easy transitioning when one decides to start.

Key principles of plant-based diet

- a lot of emphasis on whole foods and minimal focus on processed food. Always whole foods mainly are plant-based while processed food mostly comprises of animal products. A plant-based diet is high in nutrients and contains fewer calories. For this reason, even when taken in large quantities, it's not easy for someone to gain weight compared to processed foods. The ease in absorption and digestion and the extra fiber helps prevent constipation.
- focuses mostly on the plant, which includes but not limited to fruits, whole grains, vegetables, legumes, nuts, seeds, and vegetables. These should comprise the majority of the food one eats, and one should very strict enough to follow the diet. All serving should contain more plants and less animal protein to enjoy the full benefits.

- quality is more important than quantity; by this, i mean fresh, locally available, or organic is healthier and nutritious. You can liaise with local farmers and get fresh farm produce and prepare at home. Fresh from the farm is more nutritious and very tasty. Green vegetables lose their nutrients with time if not appropriately stored; thus, should be cooked while still green.
- always consume fats that are healthy, avoid refined fats and oil processed with lots of chemicals. Go for unsaturated fats, which are very good and healthy for your heart. Unhealthy fats are hard to absorb and sometimes bring some health risks like blocked arteries and diabetes.
- start your plant-based with breakfast because this is the meal no one would think should have any vegetables at all. You can take fruit salad; add spinach or kale to your eggs or cauliflower smoothie. Healthy breakfast every morning is crucial and should be taken with seriousness, especially if one has started a vegetarian diet. It will give your body the energy needed to start and go through the day, thus making your brain active throughout the day.
- experiment with at least one plant every week. It will increase the variety of vegetables you're used to every week.

Additionally, it will also boost your nutrient every week but also make you have a variety to choose from, thus reducing restrictions.

It will also expose you to a big world of the various plant-based meal and categorize them as in, easy to prepare, favorite, most nutritious, and tastier.

Those who love meat and fast food often struggle when they start a plant-based diet and can sometimes even find it annoying. Doctors will recommend reducing animal protein intake and maximizing on plants, but how many times have we ignored doctors' recommendations? It's not comfortable with the current fast-paced life, which gives no time to prepare a home-cooked meal.

Also, some people stay places far away from farmers or where access to fresh farm produce is not easy; however, there are some tips you can use so that you don't run out of stock and start indulging. You can buy groceries in bulk worth one week and ensure you store them properly. Poor storage can spoil them, thus making them not suitable for human consumption.

Compared to fast and processed food, plant-based meals can be slightly expensive, that's why some people may be tempted to grab fast food during lunch, which is cheaper and readily available. It is thus useful to look at long term benefits, potential risks, and your state of health. The cost of medication is or maybe even more expensive than plants and vegetables. This long-term benefit makes it worth investing in plant-based meals, which are fresh, nutritious, and healthy.

Kindly keep in mind that people who have some of the diseases discussed above are not vegetarian, and this plant-based meal will not prevent one from getting those diseases, but the diet lowers the risk. Your doctor needs to give you consent if you're on medication or if you have some allergies or just for the doctor to provide you with the approval that it's okay to start a plant-based meal.

Some people are allergic to some grains or nuts; you can get an alternative that is healthy and has the same of better nutritional value. The plant should be included from the first meal of the day, which is breakfast. Include as much as you possibly can, make it appetizing and appealing, if you don't know where to start from do not worry since the next chapters have some simple yet effective recipes that you can use. The recipes contain breakfast, lunch, and supper.

If you are doing a plant-based meal for health reasons, bring your family on board if possible, let them know why you have decided to change your eating habit. Chances are, they will be very appreciative and would give the necessary moral support that you need, you'll also be helping them as they will also consume healthy plant meals, thus live healthier fulfilling lives.

Family and friends can also give recommendations on where to get fresh produce; they can motivate and encourage one another.

Eating plant-based meals will help you realize a healthy lifestyle. Thus, healthy living; people who live healthy lives, have more fulfilling, and rewarding lives, therefore, they are happier content, and less anxious. They are also active and not conscious of their bodies since they are rarely overweight.

Not all plant-based meal is healthy the same way as not all animal protein is harmful. So, as you embark on a plant-based meal, confirm and recheck the quality and nutritional values. The best part about a plant-based diet is the low-calorie rate and less fatty. Ensure that you take the recommended calories without overindulging or depriving yourself.

The best news with a plant-based diet is you are not permanently restricted from taking animal protein, but you can choose it in very minimal quantities. This is good news for animal protein lovers and makes the meal plan workable and worth trying. The diet is also progressive in the sense that you can start slowly and not necessarily cutting on all animal protein intake at ago.

Health workers are currently encouraging people who are not sick to eat healthy so as to boost their immunity and help their body be able to fight some pathogens without medication. It is also interesting to note that medicines are made using herbs and some plants. Why wait to be sick if a plant-based meal can prevent some sickness?

Plant-based meal, therefore, is an essential diet, and if everyone can get started, then we can have a very healthier nation. It is one of the most inclusive vegetarian related diets. Different places have different plants depending on the season so you can take advantage of the season and purchase fresh and locally produced and enjoy the raw nutrients.

Also, one can link with local farmers and ensure that you get quality for your money or instead of purchasing immediately it's got from the farm and prepare the same day, thus preserving the nutrients. A plant-based meal is not easy but realistic and doable as long as you put your mind to it. Redefine yourself today and start consuming a plant-based diet.

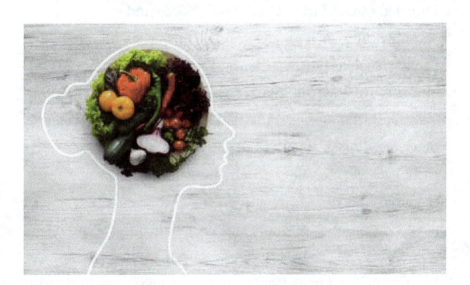

Chapter 3: 5 Reasons to Follow A Plant-Based Diet for Weight Loss

Plant based diet isn't an automatic ticket to lose weight. Come to think of it: you didn't gain the weight in one day so how do you think you will lose the weight immediately?

With consistency, discipline and a lot of work, you can lose weight while you're on the plant-based diet. Here are a few tips that can help you

Eat the three most important meals of the day

Breakfast, lunch and dinner are the most important meals of the day and you should try not to skip them. These three meals should consist of whole foods with almost no processing. Go for whole grain foods, vegetables and beans. Forget about all forms of processed foods and carbohydrates such as sugar and all forms of white flour product such as pies, cookies and cakes.

Consume only whole grain foods

Some people don't understand that there is a wide difference between whole grains (on the one hand) and processed carbohydrate, complex carbohydrate and simple sugar (on the other hand).

Some good examples of whole grains include quinoa, millet and brown rice. There are some cracked grains that are healthy too but it is better to reduce the processed grain to the barest minimum if you want to lose weight.

Stick with whole grains if you are bent on losing weight and keep out the unnecessary carbs and sugars. Studies have proven that eating whole grain foods and cereals can help you lose belly fat. So, ditch the bread and opt for oats, quinoa and other plant-based foods.

Practice portion control

Whether you are eating plant-based diet or whole grain foods, portion control is the way to go. You can't eat 5 different heavy dishes of whole grain foods and expect to lose weight. Two slices of bread made from wheat or barley or a less than 7 tablespoon of oats is enough for breakfast. Drinks lots of water to encourage metabolism and avoid eating in between meals as much as you can.

Up legumes, down carbs

Take more legumes, beans and beans products and eat it once in a day. You can eat it twice a day if you don't mind it. Eat beans and legumes in the place of carbs.

Beans with little or no oil content are pretty rich in fiber and other nutrients but low in fat. Even though many people don't believe it, if you take lots of beans and chew them properly, you will actually you will get the protein value with little or no fat or calories.

You can try out canned beans but try cooking the beans by yourself from the scratch. Good examples of legumes are black beans, tempeh, chickpeas, lentils and tofu.

Let vegetables be friends to your taste buds

Leafy greens, ground veggies, roots and plant spices and every kind of veggies you can think of should be your best friend. This is because they are low in fat and rich in fiber, nutrients and other vitamins. They will keep you full for longer and make you feel satisfied.

Little oil or no oil at all

Many people don't believe we can live without oil but we can; we are humans and we can survive without so many things. When cooking use very little amount of oil. I have had to cook for 2 weeks without using oil and i noticed reduction in my weight.

If you go on the two-week fast from oil, don't be in a hurry to go back to the oils. Reduce your oil consumption and use oils that are low in calories and high in nutrients such as olive oil, sesame oil, and extra virgin olive oil.

You can use oil for sautéing and only use 1/8 of your teaspoon to measure the amount of oil you need. You can substitute broth or water to sauté your meal.

To sauté your meals, use nuts, low-fat flax seeds, pumpkin seeds, almond seeds and nuts. You can also use seeds as toppings for your grains, cereals and brown rice.

P.s. Think of creative ways to enjoy your meal without oil.

Stop snacking

As much as you can, you need to step away from snacking on cookies but focus on fruits especially water-based fruits such as apples, berries and pears. You can have some vegetables as snacks too.

Eat early

As much as you can try to eat your dinner early; i usually recommend that you at least 2 to 3 hours before you sleep at night. Chewing slowly only helps you eat better and it tells you when you are satiated.

Plant based diet and fitness

What is healthy feeding without any consideration for fitness? These two must work together. This means you must also think of adding fitness to your lifestyle and regimen. Don't think of doing one without the other because it will help you live better and longer.

Start small

Just as you began the plant-based diet (or any new endeavor) don't push yourself too hard. It always feels like you can push yourself the extra mile and carry out a few more routines than you did the previous day. I advise that you begin with baby feet and grow.

This means you begin with a few steps and when your body is used to it, you expand your comfort zone. If you're carrying out 5 sit ups at the beginning, don't increase it to 10 the following day or 15 within the same week. Try to do the 5 sit ups for one week and then increase it to 7 or 8 by the following week.

According to habit changing research, more people are likely to make changes when they don't over strain their willpower. In case you don't know your willpower is meant to be trained or you will not know how to use it because it is weak.

You may be in need of more calories

There has been a certain perception that athletes are in need of protein; this notion has been passed by various coaches and from one coach to another.

Even though this is a myth and it isn't entirely true, many coaches, dieticians and plant-based doctors can attest to the fact that even though athletes need more calories than non-athletes because of the amount of physical energy they spend, it is a sign to take plant-based foods.

This is because consuming plant-based foods will automatically increase the level of protein you consume. All foods gotten from plants have protein in them in varying quantities but they still contain protein.

If you really need the calories there are whole plant foods that are nutritionally and calorie dense. Some of them are sweet potatoes. Avocados, seeds, beans, and nuts which are the favorites of some plant-based diet athletes.

So, if you want to get enough calories without any effect on your health, you may opt for sporting nutrition products.

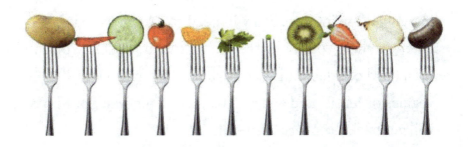

Energize yourself for workout

If you just began to work out you wouldn't need any to energize yourself by taking on more calories for the better part of your work out.

When your regimen increases or if you begin to carry out high intensity exercises, especially if the duration of the workout is more than one hour, you'll notice that you get burnt out really quickly.

This means you need to eat something to serve as a replacement for the energy you are burning during the duration of the exercise.

Another good fruit that can energize you for your workout is medjool dates. You can take out the pits and eat brazil nuts. There are quick and healthy sources of whole plant-based food calories. There are quite a number of seeds, nuts and fruits that helps your body to be strong enough to go through the motions of working out.

Whenever your workout spans for longer period or hours and if it gets more intense, you will need to take in enough energy to help your body recover all that it has lost. You can try a bowl of salad and beans, whole grain pasta with veggies or lentils and any quinoa meal. This way, your body will get back the energy it burnt.

Stay hydrated always

As you work out, you'll notice that you sweat; this means that you are losing fluids. You need to take in more fluids to replace the fluid you lost.

So how much fluid should you take?

If you understand your body quite well, you'll know when you're dehydrated. If your work out isn't too long, you'll be fine just taking a little water. You can try to take 4 to 6 ounces of water within 10 to 20 minutes while you're exercising.

If you have to work out for long periods at a stretch (may be about 2 to 3 hours if you have to run a marathon, or if you sweat a lot you can pour some electrolytes to your water so as to prevent hyponatremia.

Hyponatremia is a critical condition that is linked to over hydration. For shorter workout exercises, you can take can take more fruits because they have potassium and sodium. You can also add a pinch of salt to the sports drink you make yourself so it will balance the levels of your electrolyte.

Rest! Rest! Rest!

I can't emphasize this enough, rest is important. When you rest properly, you give your body time to recover. You burn out a part of yourself when you work out and you need to recover.

Many people forget that this is important and i don't blame anyone since i'm also guilty of doing this; we are always in a hurry because it seems 24 hours is not enough. Rest is important.

This is where it gets interesting; plant-based diet have anti-inflammatory contents and they are nutritionally dense whole plant foods that can help you to recover as quickly as possible.

This is why you can need to give yourself time before you pour yourself into other things. There's nothing wrong with working out every day; without proper rest it will affect the other things you daily even to talking with others, sex or any light activity you try to insert yourself.

Don't forget to get the required sleep you need in a day; sleep helps your body and mind to rest. This will strengthen the body in preparation for the next day. Try taking a nap in the afternoon and you'll see how refreshed you feel when you wake up.

You deserve your rest so take it.

Chapter 4: What to Eat and What to Avoid

Foods to eat

Fruits. Berries would be the yummiest foods about the plant-based diet, as they feature lots of all-natural sugars. As soon as your taste buds start to recover from all of the sugar, then you'll have the ability to taste as much sweetness out of a banana because most men and women flavor in their ice cream or banana cream pie.

Vegetables. Vegetables, particularly leaf veggies are thought to be among the healthiest foods on the planet. On the other hand, the single thing with leaf veggies is they are sometimes bitter, and might not be attractive when you transition into the plant diet.

Herbs. Herbs can also be sour, but as with leaf vegetables they're quite beneficial for you, and may even be utilized for medicinal purposes.

Nuts. Nuts are high in protein and protein additional wholesome fats, and so they're an excellent substitute for meat. You may add nuts together with the remainder of your meals, or you'll be able to take them together in a little bag or jar and bite on them between your meals.

Foods to avoid

When following a plant-based diet, highly processed foods should be avoided, and animal products minimized.

Herbal diet for detoxification and weight loss

Research has shown the tremendous impact that cellulose can have on a diet. The recommended daily dose is at least 30 years.

Cellulose is a strong, thick, and flexible fiber that gives the fruits and vegetables structural integrity. It is the main part of the plant cell - up to 70% of the plant mass consists of cellulose, which contains more than half the amount of carbon in the biosphere.

It belongs to the fiber group, which also includes pectin, lignin, gelatin, and mucous membranes.

The daily portion in a plant-based diet should be 1,000-150 kcal for women and 1,500 kcal for men, in combination with at least 30 g of cellulose.

The main foods that can be consumed are lentils, baked potatoes, beans, corn, pasta, and bread made from standard flour. Salad vegetables, as well as any fresh and dried fruits - also.

It is good to rely on low-calorie and pulp-rich vegetables. Such are tomatoes, lettuce, cauliflower, asparagus, broccoli, cucumbers, and peppers.

Other foods rich in cellulose, such as cornflakes, nuts, and dried fruits, should also be included in the menu. They supply the body with 200 kcal and 15 g of cellulose.

Chapter 5: Breakfast and Smoothies

Green Breakfast Smoothie

Preparation time: 10 minutes

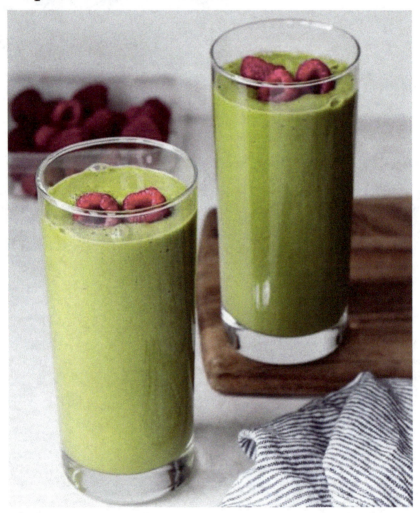

Cooking time: 0 minutes
Servings: 2

Ingredients:

- ½ banana, sliced
- 2 cups spinach or other greens, such as kale
- 1 cup sliced berries of your choosing, fresh or frozen
- 1 orange, peeled and cut into segments
- 1 cup unsweetened nondairy milk
- 1 cup ice

Directions:

Preparing the ingredients. In a blender, combine all the ingredients.

Starting with the blender on low speed, begin blending the smoothie, gradually increasing blender speed until smooth. Serve immediately.

Calories: 252, fats: 11g, carbohydrates: 21g, proteins: 14g

Blueberry Lemonade Smoothie

Preparation time: 5 minutes
Cooking time: 0 minutes
Servings: 1

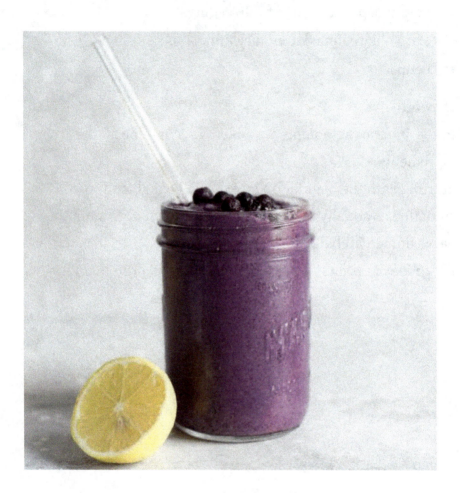

Ingredients:
- 1 cup roughly chopped kale
- ¾ cup frozen blueberries

- 1 cup unsweetened soy or almond milk
- Juice of 1 lemon
- 1 tablespoon maple syrup

Directions:

Preparing the ingredients.

Combine all the ingredients in a blender and blend until smooth. Enjoy immediately.

Calories: 122, fats: 11g, carbohydrates: 21g, proteins: 14g

Berry Protein Smoothie

Preparation time: 5 minutes
Cooking time: 0 minutes
Servings: 1

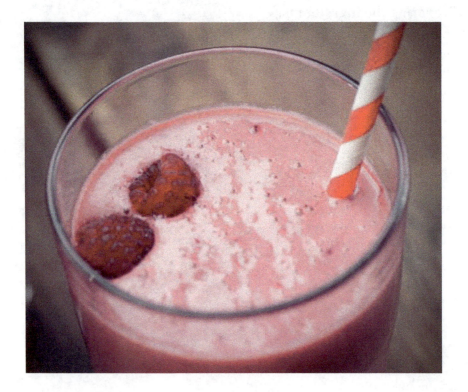

Ingredients:

- 1 banana
- 1 cup fresh or frozen berries
- ¾ cup water or nondairy milk, plus more as needed
- 1 scoop plant-based protein powder, 3 ounces silken tofu, ¼ cup rolled oats, or ½ cup cooked quinoa

Additions:

- 1 tablespoon ground flaxseed or chia seeds
- 1 handful fresh spinach or lettuce, or 1 chunk cucumber
- Coconut water to replace some of the liquid

Directions:

Preparing the ingredients

In a blender, combine the banana, berries, water, and your choice of protein.

Add any addition ingredients as desired. Purée until smooth and creamy, about 50 seconds.

Add a bit more water if you like a thinner smoothie.

Nutrition: calories: 332; protein: 7g; total fat: 5g; saturated fat: 1g; carbohydrates: 72g; fiber: 11g

Blueberry and Chia Smoothie

Preparation time: 10 minutes
Cooking time: 0 minutes
Servings: 2

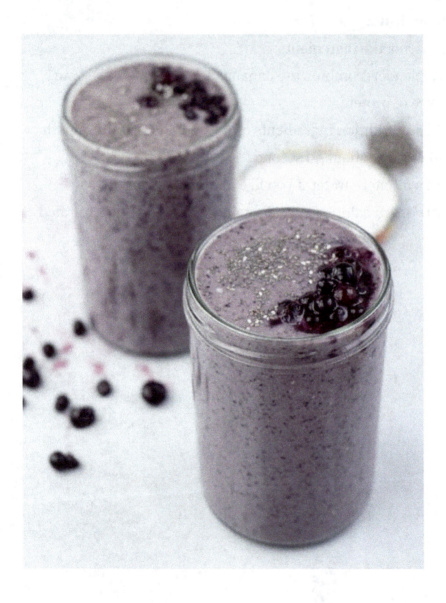

Ingredients:
- 2 tablespoons chia seeds
- 2 cups unsweetened nondairy milk
- 2 cups blueberries, fresh or frozen
- 2 tablespoons pure maple syrup or agave
- 2 tablespoons cocoa powder

Directions:

Preparing the ingredients

Soak the chia seeds in the almond milk for 5 minutes.

In a blender, combine the soaked chia seeds, almond milk, blueberries, maple syrup, and cocoa powder and blend until smooth. Serve immediately.

Calories: 200, fats: 11g, carbohydrates: 21g, proteins: 14g

Lettuce Mix Green Shake

Preparation time: 5 minutes
Cooking time: 0 minutes
Servings: 1

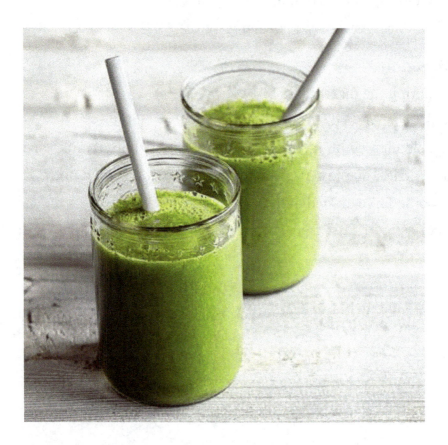

Ingredients:

- ¾ cup whole milk yogurt
- 2 cups 5-lettuce mix salad greens
- 1 packet stevia, or more to taste
- 1 tbsp mct oil

- 1 tbsp chia seeds
- 1 ½ cups water

Directions:

Add all ingredients in blender.

Blend until smooth and creamy.

Serve and enjoy.

Nutrition:

Calories: 320; carbohydrates: 19.1g; protein: 10.4g; fat: 24.2g; sugar: 9.6g; sodium: 126mg; fiber: 7.1g 56.

Basil and Pine Nuts Shake

Preparation time: 5 minutes
Cooking time: 0 minutes
Servings: 1

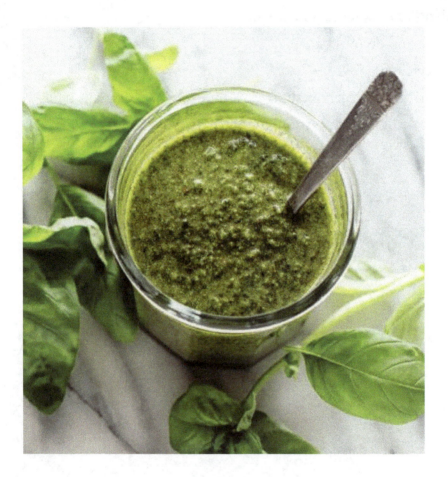

Ingredients:

- ½ cup whole milk yogurt
- 1 cup spring mix salad greens
- 1 packet stevia, or more to taste

- 1 tbsp olive oil
- 2 tbsps pine nuts, chopped
- 2 tbsps walnuts, chopped
- 10 basil leaves
- 1 tbsp hemp seeds
- 1 ½ cups water

Directions:

Add all ingredients in blender.

Blend until smooth and creamy.

Serve and enjoy.

Nutrition:

Calories: 465; carbohydrates: 14.6g; protein: 11.6g; fat: 43.2g; sugar: 7.4g; sodium: 81mg; fiber: 3.5g 57.

Rosemary-Lemon Garden Greens Smoothie

Preparation time: 5 minutes
Cooking time: 0 minutes
Servings: 1

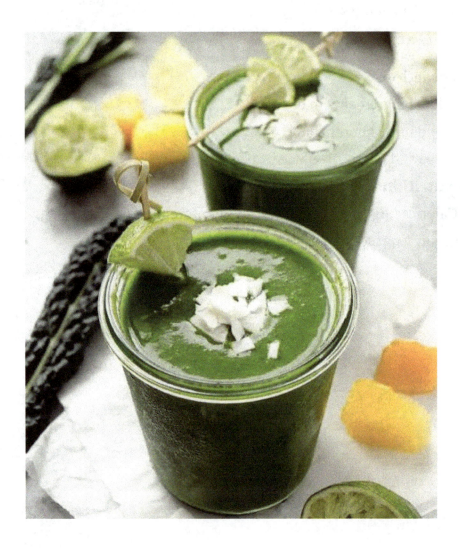

Ingredients:
- ½ cup whole milk yogurt
- 1 cup garden greens
- 1 packet stevia, or more to taste
- 1 tbsp olive oil
- 1 stalk fresh rosemary
- 1 tbsp lemon juice, fresh
- 1 tbsp pepitas
- 1 tbsp flaxseed, ground
- 1 ½ cups water

Directions:

Add all ingredients in blender.

Blend until smooth and creamy.

Serve and enjoy.

Nutrition:

Calories: 312; carbohydrates: 14.7g; protein: 9.7g; fat: 25.9g; sugar: 8.6g; sodium: 75mg; fiber: 4g *58*.

Lemon-Cilantro Greens Shake

Preparation time: 5 minutes
Cooking time: 0 minutes
Servings: 1

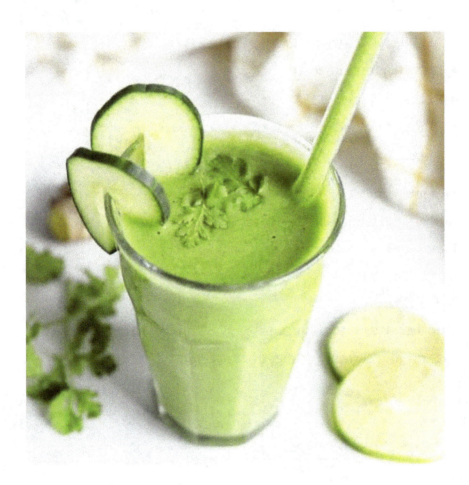

Ingredients:

- ½ cup whole milk yogurt
- 1 cup baby kale greens
- 1 packet stevia, or more to taste

- 1 tbsp avocado oil
- 1 tbsp lemon juice, fresh
- 1 tsp cilantro, chopped
- ¼ avocado fruit
- 1 tbsp flaxseed, ground
- 1 ½ cups water

Directions:

Add all ingredients in blender.

Blend until smooth and creamy.

Serve and enjoy.

Nutrition:

Calories: 345; carbohydrates: 16.4g; protein: 7.9g; fat: 29.9g; sugar: 6.9g; sodium: 76mg; fiber: 6.8g 59.

Blackberry-Chocolate Shake

Preparation time: 5 minutes
Cooking time: 0 minutes
Servings: 1

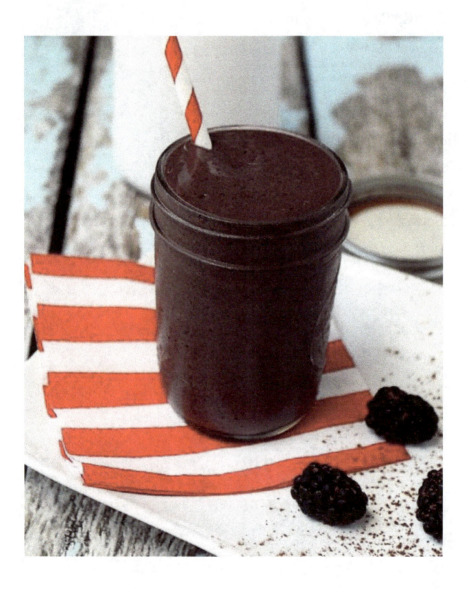

Ingredients:

- ½ cup whole milk yogurt
- ¼ cup blackberries
- 1 packet stevia, or more to taste
- 1 tbsp mct oil
- 1 tbsp dutch-processed cocoa powder
- 2 tbsps macadamia nuts, chopped
- 1 ½ cups water

Directions:

Add all ingredients in blender.

Blend until smooth and creamy.

Serve and enjoy.

Nutrition:

Calories: 463; carbohydrates: 17.9g; protein: 8.5g; fat: 43.9g; sugar: 9.1g; sodium: 67mg; fiber: 6.8g 6o.

Strawberry-Coconut Shake

Preparation time: 5 minutes
Cooking time: 0 minutes
Servings: 1

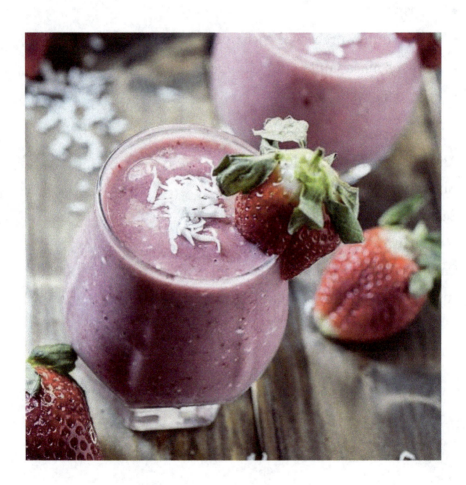

Ingredients:

- ½ cup whole milk yogurt
- 1 packet stevia, or more to taste
- 1 tbsp mct oil

- ¼ cup strawberries, chopped
- 1 tbsp coconut flakes, unsweetened
- 1 tbsp hemp seeds
- 1 ½ cups water

Directions:

Add all ingredients in blender.

Blend until smooth and creamy.

Serve and enjoy.

Nutrition:

Calories: 282; carbohydrates: 14.0g; protein: 6.5g; fat: 23.7g; sugar: 9.6g; sodium: 80mg; fiber: 2g 61.

Berry Overload Shake

Preparation time: 5 minutes
Cooking time: 0 minutes
Servings: 1

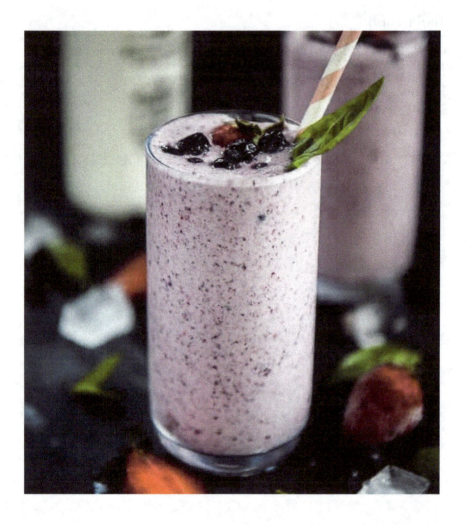

Ingredients:
- ½ cup whole milk yogurt
- 1 packet stevia, or more to taste
- ¼ cup blueberries
- ¼ cup boysenberries
- ¼ cup blackberry
- ¼ cup strawberries, chopped
- 1 tbsp avocado oil
- 1 ½ cups water

Directions:

Add all ingredients in blender.

Blend until smooth and creamy.

Serve and enjoy.

Nutrition:

Calories: 263; carbohydrates: 22.3g; protein: 5.6g; fat: 18.5g; sugar: 15.2g; sodium: 65mg; fiber: 5.3g

Mediterranean Breakfast Burrito

Preparation time: 15 minutes
Cooking time: 5 minutes
Servings: 6

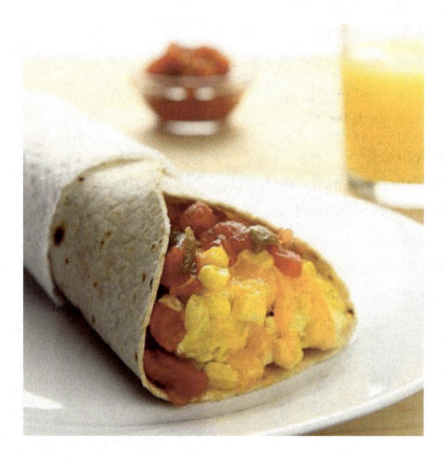

Ingredients:

- 6 tortillas whole
- 3 tbsp. Black olives
- 9 eggs

- 3 tbsp. Dried tomatoes
- 2 cup baby spinach
- ½ cup feta cheese
- ¾ cup refried beans

Directions:

Take a bowl, beat eggs and set them aside. In a nonstick pan, grease with oil and set on the medium flame. Pour the eggs batter in the and make scrambled eggs. Toss them for 5 minutes until well cooked. Add spinach, black olives, dried tomatoes and mix well. Now add the cheese and wait until cheese is melted. Pour the refried beans and wrap the eggs. Now grill the panini bread until light brown. Wrap the eggs into a panini sandwich and toss it well. Serve hot burrito

Nutrition:

Calories: 252, fats: 11g, carbohydrates: 21g, proteins: 14g

Homemade Granola

Preparation time: 5 minutes
Cooking time: 1 hour 15 minutes
Servings: 7

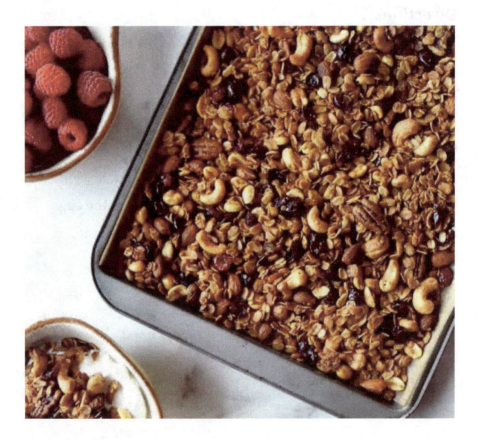

Ingredients:

- 5 cups rolled oats
- 1 cup almonds, slivered
- ¾ cup coconut, shredded
- ¾ tsp salt

- ¼ cup coconut oil
- ½ cup maple syrup

Directions:

Preheat oven to 250°f.

Mix all ingredients in a large bowl.

Spread granola evenly on two rimmed sheet pans.

Bake at 250°f for 1 hour 15 minutes, stirring every 20-25 min.

Let cool in pans, and serve.

Nutrition:

Calories 239

Fats 11 g

Carbohydrates 32 g

Protein 6 g

Breakfast Quinoa with Figs and Honey

Preparation time: 5 minutes
Cooking time: 15 minutes
Servings: 4

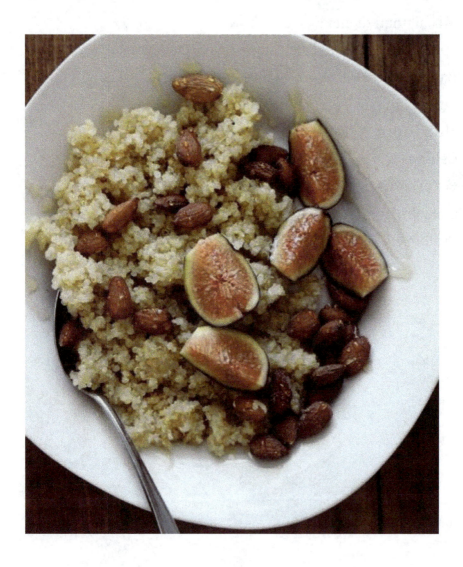

Ingredients:

- 2 cups water
- 1 cup white quinoa
- 1 cup dried figs, sliced
- 1 cup walnuts, chopped
- 1 cup almond milk
- ½ tsp cinnamon, ground
- ¼ tsp cloves, ground
- Honey, to taste

Directions:

Rinse quinoa under cool water.

Combine it with water, cinnamon, and cloves. Bring to boil.

Simmer covered for 10-15 minutes.

Add dried figs, nuts, milk. Garnish with honey. Serve.

Nutrition:

Calories 420

Carbohydrates 55 g

Fats 20 g

Protein 11 g

Maple Walnut Teff Porridge

Preparation time: 5 minutes
Cooking time: 20 minutes
Servings: 2

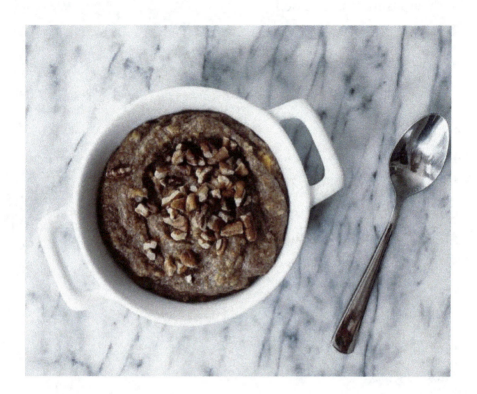

Ingredients:

- 1 ½ cups water
- 1 cup teff, whole grain
- ½ cup coconut milk
- ½ tsp cardamom, ground
- ¼ cup walnuts, chopped

- 1 tsp sea salt
- 1 tbsp maple syrup

Directions:

Combine the water and coconut oil in a medium pot. Bring to boil, then stir in the teff.

Add the cardamom, and simmer uncovered for 15-20 minutes. Mix in the maple syrup and walnuts. Serve.

Nutrition:

Calories 312

Carbohydrates 35 g

Fats 18 g

Protein 7 g

Chapter 6: Main Dishes

Black Bean Stuffed Sweet Potatoes

Preparation time: 15 minutes
Cooking time: 65 minutes
Servings: 4

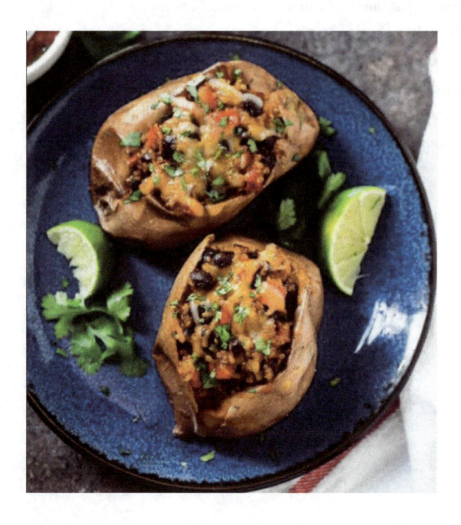

Ingredients:

- 4 large sweet potatoes
- 15 ounces cooked black beans
- 1/2 teaspoon ground black pepper
- 1/2 of a medium red onion, peeled, diced
- 1/2 teaspoon sea salt
- 1/4 teaspoon onion powder
- 1/4 teaspoon garlic powder
- 1/4 teaspoon red chili powder
- 1/4 teaspoon cumin
- 1 teaspoon lime juice
- 1 1/2 tablespoons olive oil
- 1/2 cup cashew cream sauce

Directions:

Spread sweet potatoes on a baking tray greased with oil and bake for 65 minutes at 350 degrees f until tender.

Meanwhile, prepare the sauce, and for this, whisk together the cream sauce, black pepper and lime juice until combined, set aside until required.

When 10 minutes of the baking time of potatoes are left, heat a skillet pan with oil, then add onion and cook for 5 minutes until golden.

Then stir in spice, cook for another 3 minutes, stir in bean until combined and cook for 5 minutes until hot.

Let roasted sweet potatoes cool for 10 minutes, then cut them open, mash the flesh and top with bean mixture, cilantro and avocado, and then drizzle with cream sauce.

Serve straight away.

Nutrition:

Calories: 387

Fat: 16.1 g

Carbs: 53 g

Protein: 10.4 g

Fiber: 17.6 g

Black Bean and Quinoa Salad

Preparation time: 10 minutes
Cooking time: 0 minute
Servings: 10

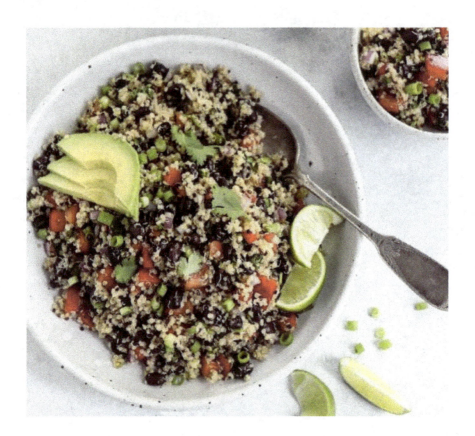

Ingredients:

- 15 ounces cooked black beans
- 1 medium red bell pepper, cored, chopped
- 1 cup quinoa, cooked
- 1 medium green bell pepper, cored, chopped

- 1/2 cup vegan feta cheese, crumbled

Directions:

Place all the ingredients in a large bowl, except for cheese, and stir until incorporated.

Top the salad with cheese and serve straight away.

Nutrition:

Calories: 64

Fat: 1 g

Carbs: 8 g

Protein: 3 g

Fiber: 3 g

Grilled Zucchini with Tomato Salsa

Preparation time: 10 minutes
Cooking time: 8 minutes
Servings: 4

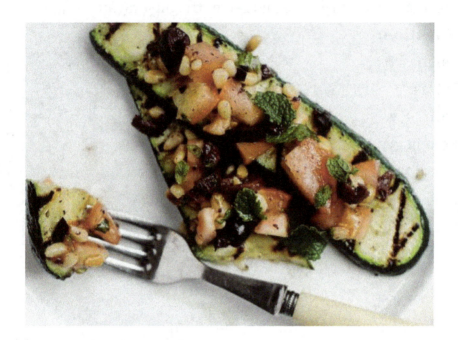

Ingredients:

- 4 zucchinis, sliced
- 1 tbsp. Olive oil
- Salt and pepper to taste
- 1 cup tomatoes, chopped
- 1 tbsp. Mint, chopped
- 1 tsp. Red wine vinegar

Directions:

- Preheat your grill.
- Coat the zucchini with oil and season with salt and pepper.
- Grill for 4 minutes per side.
- Mix the remaining ingredients in a bowl.
- Top the grilled zucchini with the minty salsa.

Nutritional value:

Calories 71

Total fat 5 g

Saturated fat 1 g

Cholesterol 0 mg

Sodium 157 mg

Total carbohydrate 6 g

Dietary fiber 2 g

Protein 2 g

Total sugars 4 g

Potassium 413 mg

Eggplant Parmesan

Preparation time: 20 minutes
Cooking time: 1 hour
Servings: 8

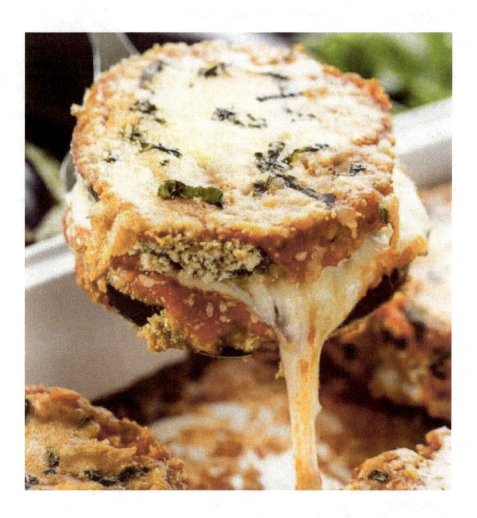

Ingredients:

- Cooking spray
- 2 eggplants, sliced into rounds
- Salt and pepper to taste
- 2 tbsp. Olive oil
- 1 cup onion, chopped
- 2 cloves garlic, crushed and minced
- 28 oz. Crushed tomatoes
- ¼ cup red wine
- 1 tsp. Dried basil
- 1 tsp. Dried oregano
- ½ cup parmesan cheese
- 1 cup mozzarella cheese
- Basil leaves, chopped

Directions:

Preheat your oven to 400 degrees f.

Spray your baking pan with oil.

Arrange the eggplant in the baking pan.

Season with salt and pepper.

Roast for 20 minutes.

In a pan over medium heat, add the oil and cook the onion for 4 minutes.

Add the garlic and cook for 1 to 2 minutes.

Stir in the rest of the ingredients except the cheese and basil.

Simmer for 10 minutes.

Spread the sauce on a baking dish.

Top with the eggplant slices.

Sprinkle the mozzarella and parmesan on top.

Bake in the oven for 25 minutes.

Nutritional value:

Calories 192

Total fat 9 g

Saturated fat 4 g

Cholesterol 18 mg

Sodium 453 mg

Total carbohydrate 16 g

Dietary fiber 5 g

Protein 10 g

Total sugars 8 g

Potassium 632 mg

Coconut Chickpea Curry

Preparation time: 10 minutes
Cooking time: 30 minutes
Servings: 4

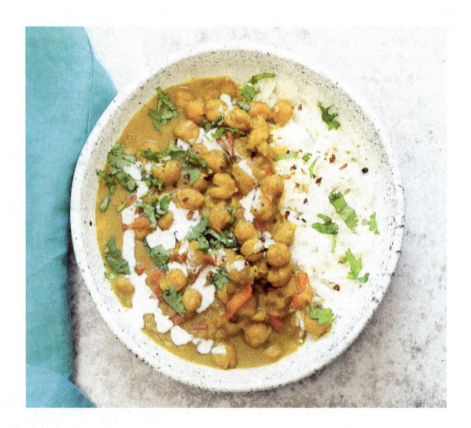

Ingredients:

- 2 teaspoons coconut flour
- 16 ounces cooked chickpeas
- 14 ounces tomatoes, diced
- 1 large red onion, sliced

- 1 ½ teaspoon minced garlic
- ½ teaspoon of sea salt
- 1 teaspoon curry powder
- 1/3 teaspoon ground black pepper
- 1 ½ tablespoons garam masala
- 1/4 teaspoon cumin
- 1 small lime, juiced
- 13.5 ounces coconut milk, unsweetened
- 2 tablespoons coconut oil

Directions:

Take a large pot, place it over medium-high heat, add oil and when it melts, add onions and tomatoes, season with salt and black pepper and cook for 5 minutes.

Switch heat to medium-low level, cook for 10 minutes until tomatoes have released their liquid, then add chickpeas and stir in garlic, curry powder, garam masala, and cumin until combined.

Stir in milk and flour, bring the mixture to boil, then switch heat to medium heat and simmer the curry for 12 minutes until cooked.

Taste to adjust seasoning, drizzle with lime juice, and serve.

Nutrition:

Calories: 225

Fat: 9.4 g

Carbs: 28.5 g ; Protein: 7.3 g ; Fiber: 9 g

Mediterranean Chickpea Casserole

Preparation time: 10 minutes
Cooking time: 60 minutes
Servings: 4

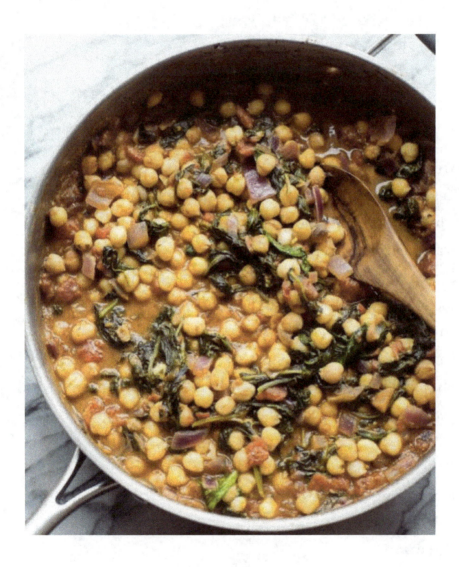

Ingredients:

- 3 cups baby spinach
- 2 medium red onions, peeled, diced
- 2 1/2 cups tomatoes
- 3 cups cooked chickpeas
- 1 ½ teaspoon minced garlic
- 1/3 teaspoon ground black pepper
- 1 ¼ teaspoon salt
- 1/4 teaspoon allspice
- 1 tablespoon coconut sugar
- 1 teaspoon dried oregano
- 1/4 teaspoon cayenne
- 1/4 teaspoon cloves
- 2 bay leaves
- 1 tablespoon coconut oil
- 2 tablespoons olive oil
- 1 cup vegetable stock
- 1 lemon, juiced
- 2 ounces vegan feta cheese

Directions:

Take a large skillet pan, place it over medium-high heat, add coconut oil and when it melts, add onion and cook for 5 minutes until softened.

Switch heat to medium-low level, stir in garlic, cook for 2 minutes, then stir in tomatoes, add all the spices and bay leaves, pour in the stock, stir until mixed and cook for 20 minutes.

Then stir in chickpeas, simmer cooking for 15 minutes until the cooking liquid has reduced by one-third, stir in spinach and cook for 3 minutes until it begins to wilt.

Then stir in olive oil, sugar and lemon juice, taste to adjust seasoning, and remove and discard bay leaves.

When done, top chickpeas with cheese, broil for 5 minutes until cheese has melted and golden brown, then garnish with parsley and serve.

Nutrition:

Calories: 257.8

Fat: 3.8 g

Carbs: 47.1 g

Protein: 10.3 g

Fiber: 9.4 g

Sweet Potato and White Bean Skillet

Preparation time: 10 minutes
Cooking time: 45 minutes
Servings: 4

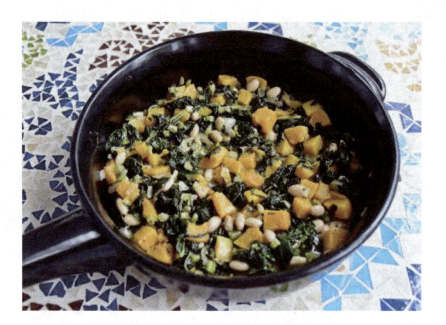

Ingredients:

- 1 large bunch of kale, chopped
- 2 large sweet potatoes, peeled, ¼-inch cubes
- 12 ounces cannellini beans
- 1 small onion, peeled, diced
- 1/8 teaspoon red pepper flakes
- 1 teaspoon salt
- 1 teaspoon cumin
- ½ teaspoon ground black pepper

- 1 teaspoon curry powder
- 1 1/2 tablespoons coconut oil
- 6 ounces coconut milk, unsweetened

Directions:

Take a large skillet pan, place it over medium heat, add ½ tablespoon oil and when it melts, add onion and cook for 5 minutes.

Then stir in sweet potatoes, stir well, cook for 5 minutes, then season with all the spices, cook for 1 minute and remove the pan from heat.

Take another pan, add remaining oil in it, place it over medium heat and when oil melts, add kale, season with some salt and black pepper, stir well, pour in the milk and cook for 15 minutes until tender.

Then add beans, beans, and red pepper, stir until mixed and cook for 5 minutes until hot.

Serve straight away.

Nutrition:

Calories: 263
Fat: 4 g
Carbs: 44 g
Protein: 13 g
Fiber: 12 g

Kung Pao Brussels Sprouts

Preparation time: 10 minutes
Cooking time: 25 minutes
Servings: 1

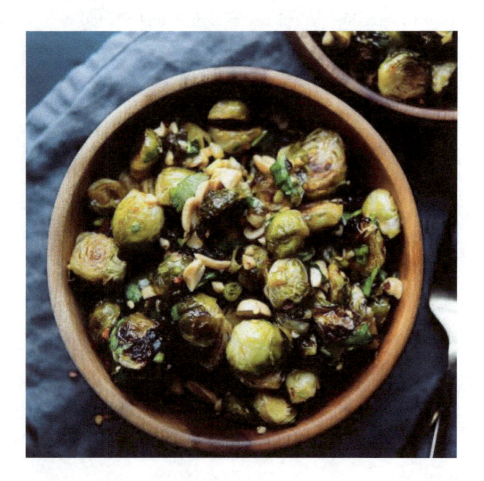

Ingredients:

- 2 pounds brussels sprouts, halved
- 1 teaspoon minced garlic
- ¾ teaspoon ground black pepper

- 1 tablespoon cornstarch
- 1 ½ teaspoon salt
- 1 tablespoon brown sugar
- 1/8 teaspoon red pepper flakes
- 1 tablespoon sesame oil
- 2 tablespoons olive oil
- 2 teaspoons apple cider vinegar
- 1/2 cup soy sauce
- 1 tablespoon hoisin sauce
- 2 teaspoons garlic chili sauce
- 1/2 cup water
- Sesame seeds as needed for garnish
- Green onions as needed for garnish
- Chopped roasted peanuts as needed for garnish

Directions:

Place sprouts on a baking sheet, drizzle with oil, season with salt and black pepper, and then bake for 20 minutes at 425 degrees f until crispy and tender.

Meanwhile, take a skillet pan, place it over medium heat, add oil and when hot, add garlic and cook for 1 minute until fragrant.

Then stir in cornstarch and remaining ingredients, except for garnishing ingredients and simmer for 3 minutes, set aside until required.

When brussel sprouts have roasted, add them to the sauce, toss until mixed and broil for 5 minutes until glazed. When done, garnish with nuts, sesame seeds, and green onions and then serve.

Nutrition:

Calories: 272

Fat: 17 g

Carbs: 26 g

Protein: 10 g

Fiber: 7 g

Balsamic-Glazed Roasted Cauliflower

Preparation time: 10 minutes
Cooking time: 1 hour and 5 minutes
Servings: 4

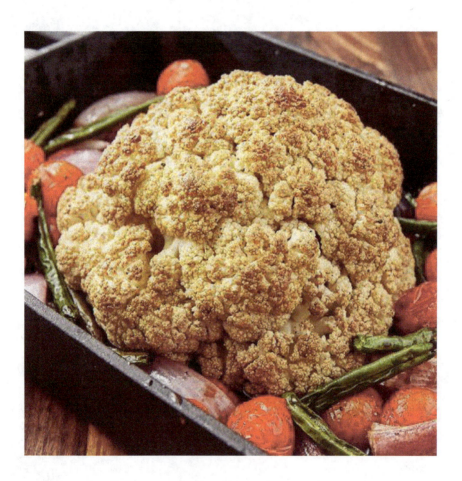

Ingredients:

- 1 large head cauliflower, cut into florets
- 1/2-pound green beans, trimmed
- 1 medium red onion, peeled, cut into wedges

- 2 cups cherry tomatoes
- ½ teaspoon salt
- 1/4 cup brown sugar
- 3 tablespoons olive oil
- 1 cup balsamic vinegar
- 2 tablespoons chopped parsley, for garnish

Directions:

Place cauliflower florets in a baking dish, add tomatoes, green beans and onion wedges around it, season with salt, and drizzle with oil.

Pour vinegar in a saucepan, stir in sugar, bring the mixture to a boil and simmer for 15 minutes until reduced by half.

Brush the sauce generously over cauliflower florets and then roast for 1 hour at 400 degrees f until cooked, brushing sauce frequently.

When done, garnish vegetables with parsley and then serve.

Nutrition:

Calories: 86

Fat: 5.7 g

Carbs: 7.7 g

Protein: 3.1 g

Fiber: 3.3 g

Stuffed Sweet Potato

Preparation time: 10 minutes
Cooking time: 45 minutes
Servings: 4

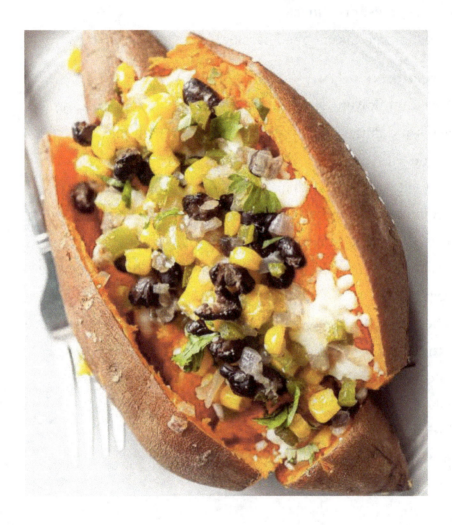

Ingredients:

- 4.5 pounds sweet potatoes
- 1/3 cup corn kernels
- 1 cup chopped kale
- 1/4 cup diced green onion
- 3/4 cup diced tomato
- ½ teaspoon minced garlic
- 1/2 teaspoon sea salt
- 1/2 teaspoon chipotle flakes
- 1/2 teaspoon dijon mustard
- 1/2 teaspoon smoked paprika
- 1/2 teaspoon liquid smoke
- 1/4 teaspoon ground turmeric
- 1/2 tablespoon lemon juice
- 3 tablespoons nutritional yeast
- 1/3 cup cashews, soaked, drained
- 1 1/2 cup pasta, cooked
- 1 cup baked pumpkin puree
- 1/2 cup vegetable broth

Directions:

Wrap each potato in a foil and then bake for 45 minutes at 375 degrees f until tender.

Meanwhile, prepare the cheese sauce and for this, place pumpkin and cashews in a food processor, add garlic, yeast, salt, paprika, chipotle flakes, liquid smoke, turmeric, mustard, and lemon juice, pour in broth and puree until smooth.

Take a pot, place it over medium-low heat, add prepared sauce, then add remaining ingredients, toss until coated, and cook for 5 minutes until kale has wilted.

Season the mixture with salt and black pepper, then switch heat to the low level and cook until sweet potatoes have roasted.

When sweet potatoes are roasted, let them stand for 10 minutes, then unwrap them, split them by slicing down the center and spoon prepared sauce generously in the center. Serve straight away.

Nutrition:

Calories: 330

Fat: 3.5 g

Carbs: 58 g

Protein: 13 g

Fiber: 15.2 g

Potatoes with Nacho Sauce

Preparation time: 10 minutes
Cooking time: 30 minutes
Servings: 4

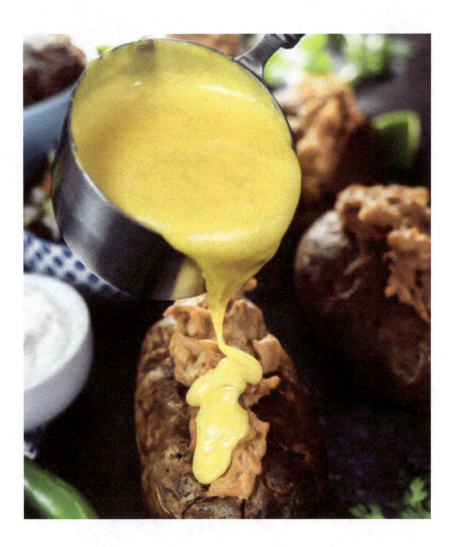

Ingredients:
- 2 pounds mixed baby potatoes, halved
- 1/2 jalapeno chili, deseeded, chopped
- 1 cup cashews, soaked, drained
- 1/2 teaspoon garlic powder
- 1/2 teaspoon red chili powder
- 1 teaspoon of sea salt
- 1/2 teaspoon sweet paprika
- 1/2 teaspoon ground cumin
- 1/4 cup nutritional yeast
- 3 tablespoons lemon juice
- 3 tablespoons olive oil
- 1 cup of water
- Tortilla chips for serving

Directions:

Place potatoes in a baking sheet, drizzle with oil, season with ½ teaspoon salt and ¼ teaspoon black pepper, and roast for 30 minutes at 450 degrees f until crispy and golden.

Meanwhile, place the remaining ingredients in a blender and pulse for 2 minutes until smooth.

Tip the sauce in a saucepan and cook for 5 minutes at the medium-low level until warm and then serve with roasted potatoes and tortilla chips.

Nutrition:

Calories: 380; Fat: 18 g ; Carbs: 47 g ; Protein: 10 g ; Fiber: 6 g

Veggie Kabobs

Preparation time: 10 minutes
Cooking time: 10 minutes
Servings: 10

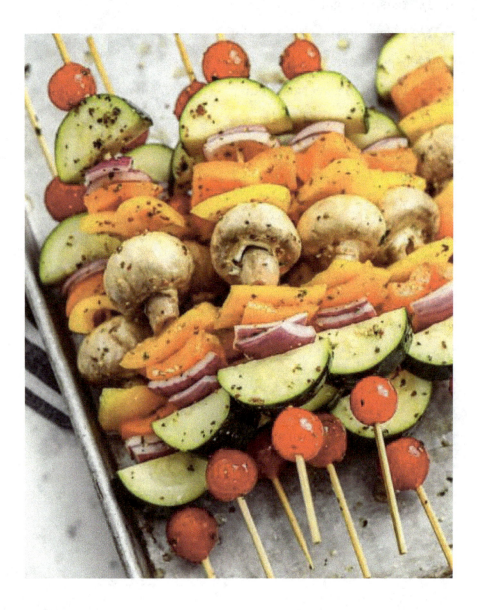

Ingredients:

- 8 ounces button mushrooms, halved
- 2 pounds summer squash, peeled, 1-inch cubed
- 12 ounces small broccoli florets
- 2 cups grape tomatoes
- 1 teaspoon salt
- 1/2 teaspoon smoked paprika
- 1 teaspoon ground cumin
- 6 tablespoons olive oil
- 1/2 teaspoon ground coriander
- 1 lime, juiced

Directions:

Toss broccoli florets with 1 tablespoon oil, toss tomatoes and squash pieces with 2 tablespoons oil, then toss mushrooms with 1 tablespoon oil and thread these vegetables onto skewers.

Grill mushrooms and broccoli for 7 to 10 minutes, squash and tomatoes and 8 minutes, and when done, transfer the skewers to a plate and drizzle with lime juice and remaining oil.

Prepared the spice mix and for this, stir together salt, paprika, cumin, and coriander, sprinkle half of the mixture over grilled veggies, cover them with foil for 5 minutes, and then sprinkle with the remaining spice mix.

Nutrition: Calories: 110; Fat: 9 g ; Carbs: 8 g ; Protein: 3 g; Fiber:

Summer Pesto Pasta

Preparation time: 10 minutes
Cooking time: 10 minutes
Servings: 4

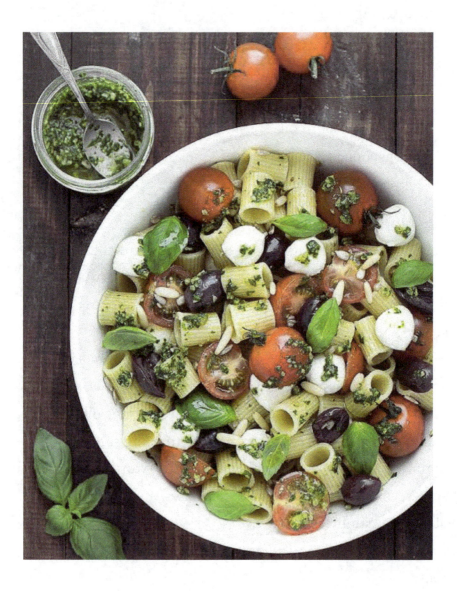

Ingredients:

- 1-pound whole-grain spaghetti, cooked
- 2 cups grape tomatoes, halved
- 2 ears corn, shucked
- 1 medium yellow squash, ½ inch sliced
- 1 small bell pepper, deseeded, cut into sixths
- 1 medium zucchini, ½ inch sliced
- 1/4 cup chopped parsley
- 4 green onions
- 1 teaspoon salt
- 1 teaspoon ground black pepper
- 1 lemon, juiced, zested
- 2 tablespoons olive oil
- 1/2 cup vegan pesto

Directions:

Place corn, onions, bell pepper, zucchini and squash in a bowl, season with ½ teaspoon each of salt and black pepper, and toss until coated.

Grill the corn for 10 minutes, and grill remaining vegetables for 6 minutes until lightly charred and when done, chop vegetables and place them in a bowl.

Place pesto in another bowl, add lemon juice and zest, season with remaining salt and black pepper, and whisk until combined.

Pour pesto over vegetables, toss until mixed, then cut kernels from grilled cobs, add them to the vegetables, then add pasta, parsley, and tomatoes and toss until combined.
Serve straight away.

Nutrition:

Calories: 370

Fat: 12 g

Carbs: 54 g

Protein: 12 g

Fiber: 5 g

Linguine with Wild Mushrooms

Preparation time: 5 minutes
Cooking time: 3 minutes
Servings: 4

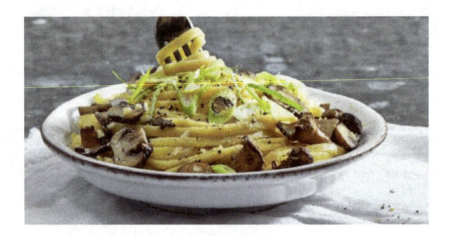

Ingredients:

- 12 ounces mixed mushrooms, sliced
- 2 green onions, sliced
- 1 ½ teaspoon minced garlic
- 1-pound whole-grain linguine pasta, cooked
- 1/4 cup nutritional yeast
- ½ teaspoon salt
- ¾ teaspoon ground black pepper
- 6 tablespoons olive oil
- ¾ cup vegetable stock, hot

Directions:

Take a skillet pan, place it over medium-high heat, add garlic and mushroom and cook for 5 minutes until tender.

Transfer the vegetables to a pot, add pasta and remaining ingredients, except for green onions, toss until combined and cook for 3 minutes until hot.

Garnish with green onions and serve.

Nutrition:

Calories: 430

Fat: 15 g

Carbs: 62 g

Protein: 15 g

Fiber: 5 g

Edamame and Noodle Salad

Preparation time: 5 minutes
Cooking time: 5 minutes
Servings: 4

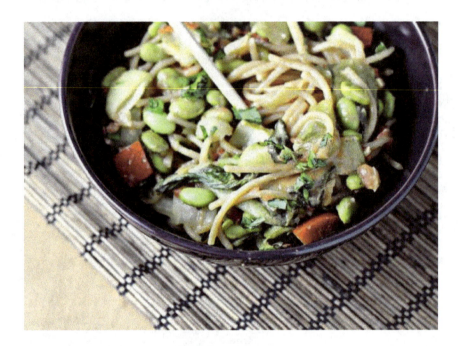

Ingredients:

- 24 ounces shirataki noodles
- 1 medium apple, sliced
- 2 cups grape tomatoes, halved
- 3 cups frozen edamame, shelled
- 3 cups shredded carrots
- 2 cups frozen corn
- 1/2 teaspoon salt

- 1/2 cup rice vinegar
- 1 tablespoon sriracha hot sauce and more for serving
- 1/2 cup peanut butter
- 2 tablespoons water
- 1/2 cup chopped cilantro

Directions:

Take a large pot, place it over high heat, pour in water, bring it to boil, then add noodles, corn and edamame, boil for 2 minutes and drain when done.

Place remaining ingredients in a large bowl, whisk until combined, then add boiled vegetables and toss until well coated.

Drizzle with more sriracha sauce and toss until combined.

Nutrition:

Calories: 455
Fat: 22 g
Carbs: 50 g
Protein: 22 g
Fiber: 13 g

Pilaf with Garbanzos and Dried Apricots

Preparation time: 10 minutes
Cooking time: 15 minutes
Servings: 4

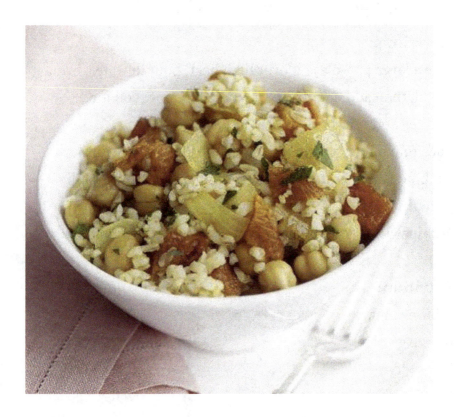

Ingredients:

- 1 cup bulgur
- 6 ounces cooked chickpeas
- 1/2 cup dried apricot
- 1 small white onion, peeled, diced
- ½ teaspoon minced garlic

- 2 teaspoons curry powder
- 1/2 teaspoon salt
- 1 tablespoon olive oil
- 1/4 cup fresh parsley leaves
- 2 cups vegetable broth
- 3/4 cup water

Directions:

Take a saucepan, place it over high heat, pour in water and 1 ½ cup broth, and bring it to a boil.

Then stir in bulgur, switch heat to medium-low level and simmer for 15 minutes until most of the liquid has absorbed.

Meanwhile, take a skillet pan, place it over medium heat, add oil and when hot, add onion, cook for 10 minutes, then stir in garlic and curry powder and cook for another minute.

Then add apricots, beans, and salt, pour in remaining broth and bring the mixture to boiling.

Remove pan from heat, fluff the bulgur with a fork, add to the onion-apricot mixture and stir until mixed.

Garnish with parsley and serve.

Nutrition:

Calories: 222

Fat: 4.5 g

Carbs: 35 g

Protein: 9.5 g

Fiber: 7 g

Avocado and Lime Bean Bowl

Preparation time: 10 minutes
Cooking time: 0 minute
Servings: 1

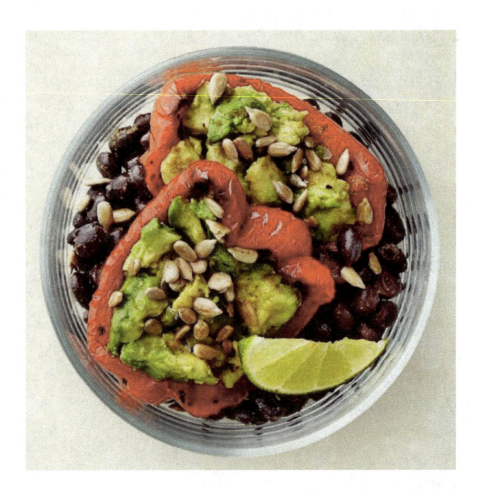

Ingredients:

- 1/2 cup mint berries
- 1/4 of medium avocado, pitted, sliced
- 1/2 cup breakfast beans
- 12 ounces roasted vegetable mix
- 1/8 teaspoon salt
- 1/8 teaspoon cumin
- 1 teaspoon sunflower seeds
- 1 teaspoon lime juice
- Lime wedges for serving

Directions:

Place avocado in a bowl, mash with a fork and then stir in lime juice, salt, and cumin until combined.

Place roasted vegetable mix in a dish, top with mashed avocado mixture, beans, and sunflower seeds.

Serve with lime wedges and berries.

Nutrition:

Calories: 292
Fat: 10.4 g
Carbs: 45.6 g
Protein: 9.7 g
Fiber: 12.1 g

Chapter 7: Soups and Stew

Sweet Potato, Corn and Jalapeno Bisque

Preparation time: 10 minutes
Cooking time: 15 minutes
Servings: 4

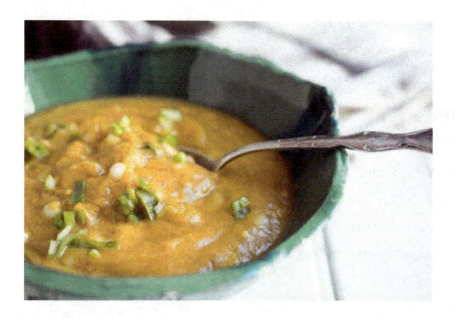

Ingredients:

- 4 ears corn
- 1 seeded and chopped jalapeno
- 4 cups vegetable broth
- 1 tablespoon olive oil
- 3 peeled and cubed sweet potatoes
- 1 chopped onion

- ½ tablespoon salt
- ¼ teaspoon black pepper
- 1 minced garlic clove

Directions:

In a pan, heat the oil over medium flame and sauté onion and garlic in it and cook for around 3 minutes. Put broth and sweet potatoes in it and bring it to boil. Reduce the flame and cook it for an additional 10 minutes. Remove it from the stove and blend it with a blender. Again, put it on the stove and add corn, jalapeno, salt, and black pepper and serve it.

Nutrition:

Carbohydrates 31g, protein 6g, fats 4g, sugar 11g.

Creamy Pea Soup with Olive Pesto

Preparation time: 20 minutes
Cooking time: 20 minutes
Servings: 4

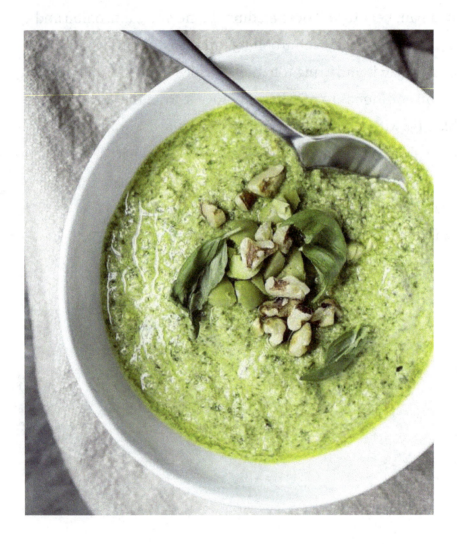

Ingredients:

- 1 grated carrot
- 1 rinsed chopped leek
- 1 minced garlic clove
- 2 tablespoons olive oil
- 1 stem fresh thyme leaves
- 15 ounces rinsed and drained peas
- ½ tablespoon salt
- ¼ teaspoon ground black pepper
- 2 ½ cups vegetable broth
- ¼ cup parsley leaves
- 1 ¼ cups pitted green olives
- 1 teaspoon drained capers
- 1 garlic clove

Directions:

Take a pan with oil and put it over medium flame and whisk garlic, leek, thyme, and carrot in it. Cook it for around 4 minutes. Add broth, peas, salt, and pepper and increase the heat. When it starts boiling, lower down the heat and cook it with a lid on for around 15 minutes and remove from heat and blend it. For making pesto whisk parsley, olives, capers, and garlic and blend it in a way that it has little chunks. Top the soup with the scoop of olive pesto.

Nutrition:

Carbohydrates 23g, protein 6g, fats 15g, sugar 4g, calories 230.

Spinach Soup with Dill and Basil

Preparation time: 10 minutes
Cooking time: 25 minutes
Servings: 8

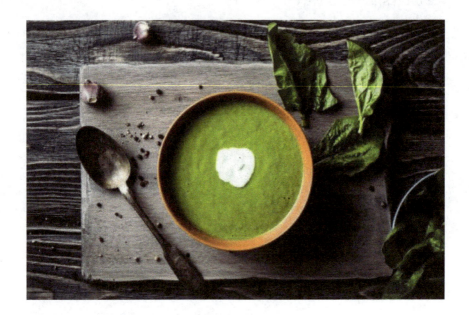

Ingredients:

- 1 pound peeled and diced potatoes
- 1 tablespoon minced garlic
- 1 teaspoon dry mustard
- 6 cups vegetable broth
- 20 ounces chopped frozen spinach
- 2 cups chopped onion
- 1 ½ tablespoons salt
- ½ cup minced dill

- 1 cup basil
- ½ teaspoon ground black pepper

Directions:

Whisk onion, garlic, potatoes, broth, mustard, and salt in a pand cook it over medium flame. When it starts boiling, low down the heat and cover it with the lid and cook for 20 minutes. Add the remaining ingredients in it and blend it and cook it for few more minutes and serve it.

Nutrition:

Carbohydrates 12g, protein 13g, fats 1g, calories 165.

Coconut Watercress Soup

Preparation time: 10 minutes
Cooking time: 20 minutes
Servings: 4

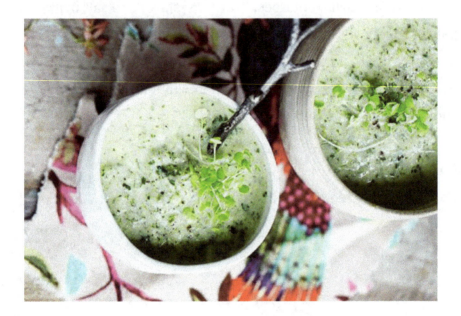

Ingredients:

- 1 teaspoon coconut oil
- 1 onion, diced
- ¾ cup coconut milk

Directions:

Preparing the ingredients.

Melt the coconut oil in a large pot over medium-high heat. Add the onion and cook until soft, about 5 minutes, then add the peas and the water. Bring to a boil, then lower the heat and add the watercress, mint, salt, and pepper.

Cover and simmer for 5 minutes. Stir in the coconut milk, and purée the soup until smooth in a blender or with an immersion blender.

Try this soup with any other fresh, leafy green—anything from spinach to collard greens to arugula to swiss chard.

Nutrition: calories: 178; protein: 6g; total fat: 10g; carbohydrates: 18g; fiber: 5g

Roasted Red Pepper and Butternut Squash Soup

Preparation time: 10 minutes
Cooking time: 45 minutes
Servings: 6

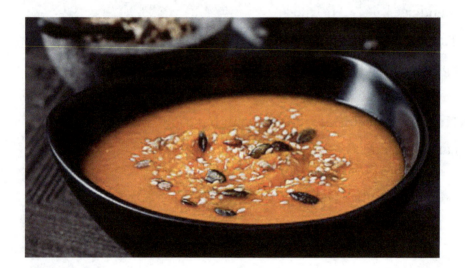

Ingredients:

- 1 small butternut squash
- 1 tablespoon olive oil
- 1 teaspoon sea salt
- 2 red bell peppers
- 1 yellow onion
- 1 head garlic
- 2 cups water, or vegetable broth
- Zest and juice of 1 lime

- 1 to 2 tablespoons tahini
- Pinch cayenne pepper
- ½ teaspoon ground coriander
- ½ teaspoon ground cumin
- Toasted squash seeds (optional)

Directions:

Preparing the ingredients.

Preheat the oven to 350°f.

Prepare the squash for roasting by cutting it in half lengthwise, scooping out the seeds, and poking some holes in the flesh with a fork. Reserve the seeds if desired.

Rub a small amount of oil over the flesh and skin, then rub with a bit of sea salt and put the halves skin-side down in a large baking dish. Put it in the oven while you prepare the rest of the vegetables.

Prepare the peppers the exact same way, except they do not need to be poked.

Slice the onion in half and rub oil on the exposed faces. Slice the top off the head of garlic and rub oil on the exposed flesh. After the squash has cooked for 20 minutes, add the peppers, onion, and garlic, and roast for another 20 minutes.

Optionally, you can toast the squash seeds by putting them in the oven in a separate baking dish 10 to 15 minutes before the vegetables are finished.

Keep a close eye on them. When the vegetables are cooked, take them out and let them cool before handling them. The squash will be very soft when poked with a fork.

Scoop the flesh out of the squash skin into a large pot (if you have an immersion blender) or into a blender.

Chop the pepper roughly, remove the onion skin and chop the onion roughly, and squeeze the garlic cloves out of the head, all into the pot or blender. Add the water, the lime zest and juice, and the tahini. Purée the soup, adding more water if you like, to your desired consistency. Season with the salt, cayenne, coriander, and cumin. Serve garnished with toasted squash seeds (if using).

Nutrition: calories: 156; protein: 4g; total fat: 7g; saturated fat: 11g; carbohydrates: 22g; fiber: 5g

Tomato Pumpkin Soup

Preparation time: 25 minutes
Servings: 4

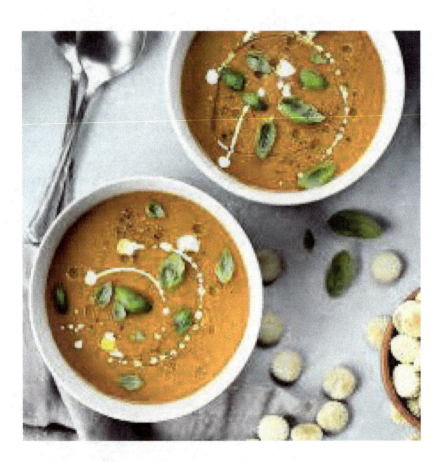

Ingredients:

- 2 cups pumpkin, diced
- 1/2 cup tomato, chopped
- 1/2 cup onion, chopped
- 1 1/2 tsp curry powder

- 1/2 tsp paprika
- 2 cups vegetable stock
- 1 tsp olive oil
- 1/2 tsp garlic, minced

Directions:

In a saucepan, add oil, garlic, and onion and sauté for 3 minutes over medium heat.

Add remaining ingredients into the saucepan and bring to boil. Reduce heat and cover and simmer for 10 minutes.

Puree the soup using a blender until smooth.

Stir well and serve warm.

Nutrition: calories 70; fat 2.7 g; carbohydrates 13.8 g; sugar 6.3 g; protein 1.9 g; cholesterol 0 mg

Cauliflower Spinach Soup

Total time: 45 minutes

Servings: 5

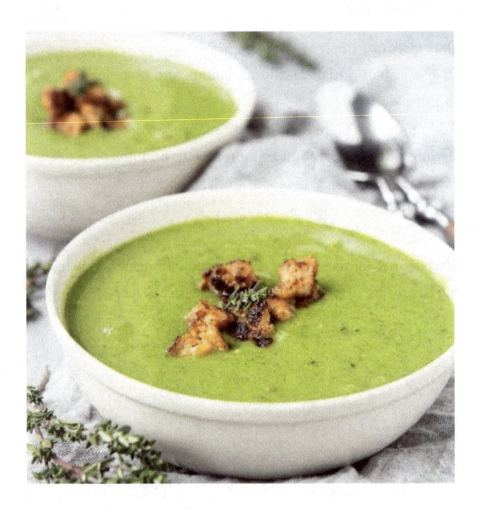

Ingredients:

- 1/2 cup unsweetened coconut milk
- 5 oz fresh spinach, chopped
- 5 watercress, chopped

- 8 cups vegetable stock
- 1 lb cauliflower, chopped
- Salt

Directions:

Add stock and cauliflower in a large saucepan and bring to boil over medium heat for 15 minutes.

Add spinach and watercress and cook for another 10 minutes. Remove from heat and puree the soup using a blender until smooth.

Add coconut milk and stir well. Season with salt.

Stir well and serve hot.

Nutritional value (amount per serving): calories 153; fat 8.3 g; carbohydrates 8.7 g; sugar 4.3 g; protein 11.9 g; cholesterol 0 mg

Avocado Mint Soup

Total time: 10 minutes

Servings: 2

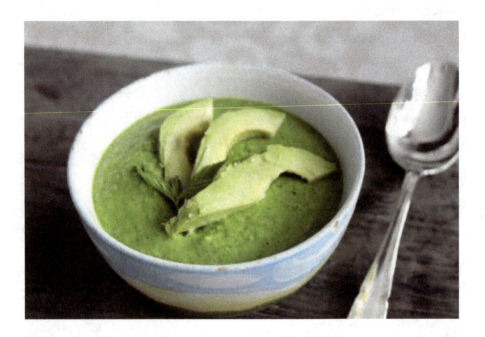

Ingredients:

- 1 medium avocado, peeled, pitted, and cut into pieces
- 1 cup coconut milk
- 2 romaine lettuce leaves
- 20 fresh mint leaves
- 1 tbsp fresh lime juice
- 1/8 tsp salt

Directions:

Add all ingredients into the blender and blend until smooth. Soup should be thick not as a puree.

Pour into the serving bowls and place in the refrigerator for 10 minutes.

Stir well and serve chilled.

Nutritional value (amount per serving): calories 268; fat 25.6 g; carbohydrates 10.2 g; sugar 0.6 g; protein 2.7 g; cholesterol 0 mg

Creamy Squash Soup

Total time: 35 minutes

Servings: 8

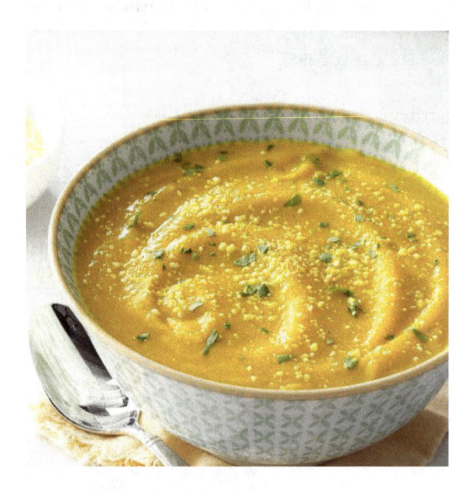

Ingredients:

- 3 cups butternut squash, chopped
- 1 ½ cups unsweetened coconut milk
- 1 tbsp coconut oil

- 1 tsp dried onion flakes
- 1 tbsp curry powder
- 4 cups water
- 1 garlic clove
- 1 tsp kosher salt

Directions:

Add squash, coconut oil, onion flakes, curry powder, water, garlic, and salt into a large saucepan. Bring to boil over high heat.

Turn heat to medium and simmer for 20 minutes.

Puree the soup using a blender until smooth. Return soup to the saucepan and stir in coconut milk and cook for 2 minutes. Stir well and serve hot.

Nutritional value (amount per serving): calories 146; fat 12.6 g; carbohydrates 9.4 g; sugar 2.8 g; protein 1.7 g; cholesterol 0 mg

Zucchini Soup

Total time: 20 minutes
Servings: 8

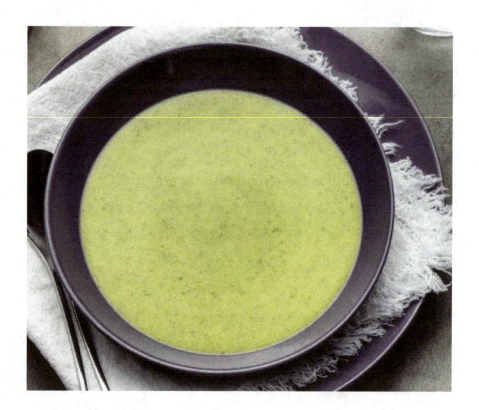

Ingredients:

- 2 ½ lbs zucchini, peeled and sliced
- 1/3 cup basil leaves
- 4 cups vegetable stock
- 4 garlic cloves, chopped
- 2 tbsp olive oil
- 1 medium onion, diced

- Pepper
- Salt

Directions:

Heat olive oil in a pan over medium-low heat.

Add zucchini and onion and sauté until softened. Add garlic and sauté for a minute.

Add vegetable stock and simmer for 15 minutes.

Remove from heat. Stir in basil and puree the soup using a blender until smooth and creamy. Season with pepper and salt.

Stir well and serve.

Nutritional value (amount per serving): calories 62; fat 4 g; carbohydrates 6.8 g; sugar 3.3 g; protein 2 g; cholesterol 0 mg

Creamy Celery Soup

Total time: 40 minutes

Servings: 4

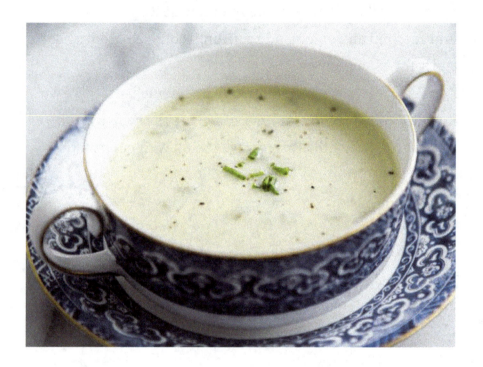

Ingredients:

- 6 cups celery
- ½ tsp dill
- 2 cups water
- 1 cup coconut milk
- 1 onion, chopped
- Pinch of salt

Directions:

Add all ingredients into the electric pot and stir well.

Cover electric pot with the lid and select soup setting.

Release pressure using a quick release method than open the lid.

Puree the soup using an immersion blender until smooth and creamy.

Stir well and serve warm.

Nutritional value (amount per serving): calories 174; fat 14.6 g; carbohydrates 10.5 g; sugar 5.2 g; protein 2.8 g; cholesterol 0 mg

Avocado Cucumber Soup

Total time: 40 minutes
Servings: 3

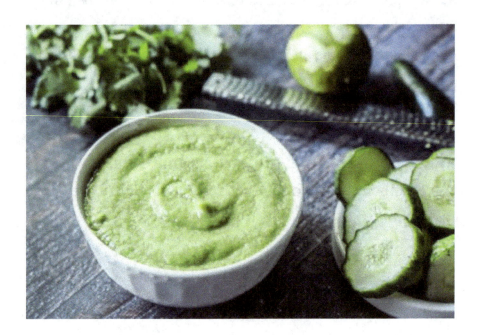

Ingredients:

- 1 large cucumber, peeled and sliced
- ¾ cup water
- ¼ cup lemon juice
- 2 garlic cloves
- 6 green onion
- 2 avocados, pitted
- ½ tsp black pepper
- ½ tsp pink salt

Directions:

Add all ingredients into the blender and blend until smooth and creamy.

Place in refrigerator for 30 minutes.

Stir well and serve chilled.

Nutritional value (amount per serving): calories 73; fat 3.7 g; carbohydrates 9.2 g; sugar 2.8 g; protein 2.2 g; cholesterol 0 mg

Garden Vegetable Stew

Preparation time: 5 minutes
Cooking time: 60 minutes
Servings: 4 servings

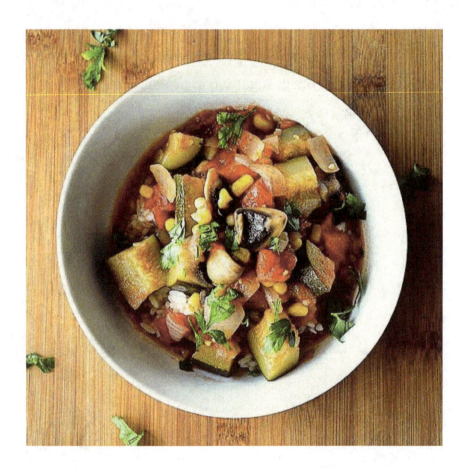

Ingredients:

- 2 tablespoons olive oil
- 1 medium red onion, chopped
- 1 medium carrot, cut into 1/4-inch slices

- ½ cup dry white wine
- 3 medium new potatoes, unpeeled and cut into 1-inch pieces
- 1 medium red bell pepper, cut into ½-inch dice
- 1½ cups vegetable broth
- 1 tablespoon minced fresh savory or 1 teaspoon dried

Directions:

1. In a large saucepan, heat the oil over medium heat. Add the onion and carrot, cover, and cook until softened, 7 minutes. Add the wine and cook, uncovered, for 5 minutes. Stir in the potatoes, bell pepper, and broth and bring to a boil. Reduce the heat to medium and simmer for 15 minutes.

2. Add the zucchini, yellow squash, and tomatoes. Season with salt and black pepper to taste, cover, and simmer until the vegetables are tender, 20 to 30 minutes. Stir in the corn, peas, basil, parsley, and savory. Taste, adjusting seasonings if necessary. Simmer to blend flavors, about 10 minutes more. Serve immediately.

Moroccan Vermicelli Vegetable Soup

Preparation time: 5 minutes

Cooking time: 35 minutes

Servings: 4 to 6 servings

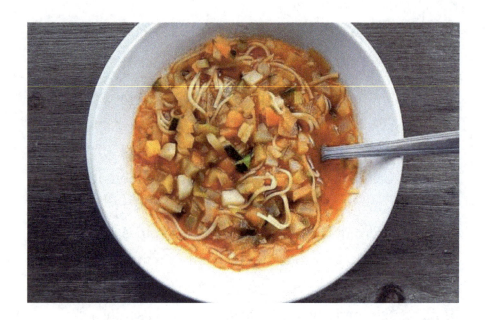

Ingredients:

- 1 tablespoon olive oil
- 1 small onion, chopped
- 1 large carrot, chopped
- 1 celery rib, chopped
- 3 small zucchini, cut into 1/4-inch dice
- 1 (28-ounce) can diced tomatoes, drained
- 2 tablespoons tomato paste

- 1½ cups cooked or 1 (15.5-ounce) can chickpeas, drained and rinsed
- 2 teaspoons smoked paprika
- 1 teaspoon ground cumin
- 1 teaspoon za'atar spice (optional)
- ¼ teaspoon ground cayenne
- 6 cups vegetable broth, homemade (see light vegetable broth) or store-bought, or water
- Salt
- 4 ounces vermicelli
- 2 tablespoons minced fresh cilantro, for garnish

Directions:

In a large soup pot, heat the oil over medium heat. Add the onion, carrot, and celery. Cover and cook until softened, about 5 minutes. Stir in the zucchini, tomatoes, tomato paste, chickpeas, paprika, cumin, za'atar, and cayenne. Add the broth and salt to taste. Bring to a boil, then reduce heat to low and simmer, uncovered, until the vegetables are tender, about 30 minutes.

Shortly before serving, stir in the vermicelli and cook until the noodles are tender, about 5 minutes. Ladle the soup into bowls, garnish with cilantro, and serve.

Moroccan Vegetable Stew

Preparation time: 5 minutes
Cooking time: 35 minutes
Servings: 4 servings

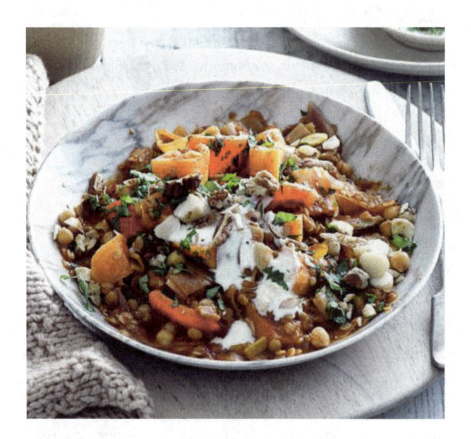

Ingredients:

- 1 tablespoon olive oil
- 2 medium yellow onions, chopped
- 2 medium carrots, cut into ½-inch dice
- ½ teaspoon ground cumin

- ½ teaspoon ground cinnamon or allspice
- ½ teaspoon ground ginger
- ½ teaspoon sweet or smoked paprika
- ½ teaspoon saffron or turmeric
- 1 (14.5-ounce) can diced tomatoes, undrained
- 8 ounces green beans, trimmed and cut into 1-inch pieces
- 2 cups peeled, seeded, and diced winter squash
- 1 large russet or other baking potato, peeled and cut into ½-inch dice
- 1½ cups vegetable broth
- 1½ cups cooked or 1 (15.5-ounce) can chickpeas, drained and rinsed
- ¾ cup frozen peas
- ½ cup pitted dried plums (prunes)
- 1 teaspoon lemon zest
- Salt and freshly ground black pepper
- ½ cup pitted green olives
- 1 tablespoon minced fresh cilantro or parsley, for garnish
- ½ cup toasted slivered almonds, for garnish

Directions:

1. In a large saucepan, heat the oil over medium heat. Add the onions and carrots, cover, and cook for 5 minutes. Stir in the cumin, cinnamon, ginger, paprika, and saffron. Cook, uncovered, stirring, for 30 seconds. Add the tomatoes, green beans, squash, potato, and broth and bring to a boil. Reduce heat to low, cover, and simmer until the vegetables are tender, about 20 minutes.

2. Add the chickpeas, peas, dried plums, and lemon zest. Season with salt and pepper to taste. Stir in the olives and simmer, uncovered, until the flavors are blended, about 10 minutes. Sprinkle with cilantro and almonds and serve immediately.

Autumn Medley Stew

Preparation time: 5 minutes
Cooking time: 60 minutes
Servings: 4 to 6 servings

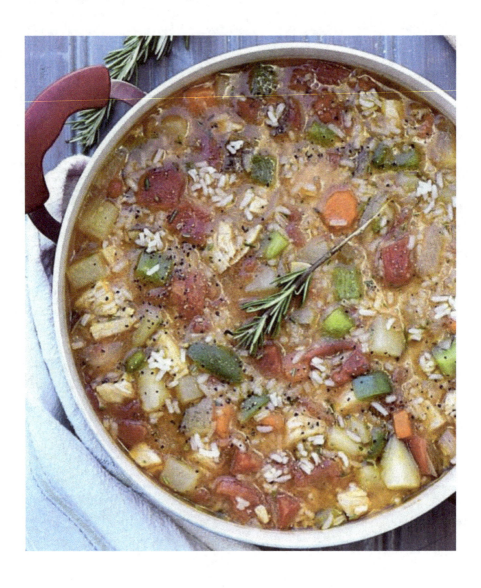

Ingredients:

- 2 tablespoons olive oil
- 8 ounces seitan, homemade or store-bought, cut in 1-inch cubes
- Salt and freshly ground black pepper
- 1 large yellow onion, chopped
- 2 garlic cloves, minced
- 1 large russet potato, peeled and cut into 1/2-inch dice
- 1 medium carrot, cut into 1/4-inch dice
- 1 medium parsnip, cut into 1/4-inch dice chopped
- 1 small butternut squash, peeled, halved, seeded, and cut into 1/2-inch dice
- 1 small head savoy cabbage, chopped
- 1 (14.5-ounce) can diced tomatoes, drained
- 1 1/2 cups cooked or 1 (15.5-ounce) can chickpeas, drained and rinsed
- 2 cups vegetable broth,
- 1/2 cup dry white wine
- 1/2 teaspoon dried marjoram
- 1/2 teaspoon dried thyme
- 1/2 cup crumbled angel hair pasta

Directions:

In a large skillet, heat 1 tablespoon of the oil over medium-high heat. Add the seitan and cook until browned on all sides, about 5 minutes. Season with salt and pepper to taste and set aside.

In a large saucepan, heat the remaining 1 tablespoon oil over medium heat. Add the onion and garlic. Cover and cook for until softened, about 5 minutes. Add the potato, carrot, parsnip, and squash. Cover and cook until softened, about 10 minutes.

Stir in the cabbage, tomatoes, chickpeas, broth, wine, marjoram, thyme, and salt and pepper to taste. Bring to a boil, then reduce heat to low. Cover and cook, stirring occasionally, until the vegetables are tender, about 45 minutes.

Add the cooked seitan and the pasta and simmer until the pasta is tender and the flavors are blended, about 10 minutes longer. Serve immediately.

Variation: leave out the pasta and serve with some warm crusty bread.

Black Bean Soup with Sweet Potato

Preparation time: 20 minutes
Cooking time: 40 minutes
Servings: 5

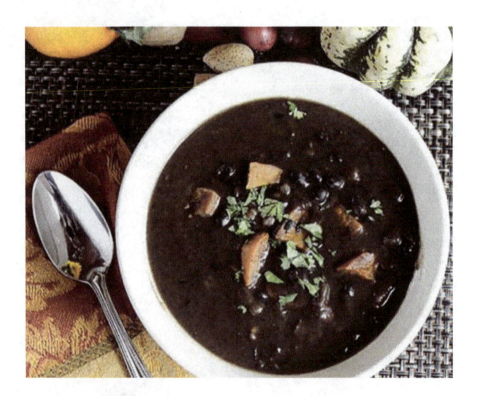

Ingredients:

- 1 ½ cups chopped onion
- 3 cups of water
- 2 teaspoons cumin seeds
- 1 ½ cups chopped red and green peppers
- ¼ teaspoon allspice

- 2 teaspoons dried oregano leaves
- ¼ teaspoon salt
- ¼ teaspoon ground black pepper
- 4 minced garlic cloves
- 2 tablespoons tomato paste
- 5 cups rinsed and drained black beans
- ¼ teaspoon red pepper flakes
- 1 tablespoon vinegar
- ½ cup diced sweet potatoes

Directions:

Whisk onion, water, pepper, black pepper, salt, oregano, cumin, red pepper flakes, all spices in a pan cook for about 7 minutes. Add garlic in it and cook for an additional one minute. After a minute, add beans, water, vinegar, and tomato paste in it and blend it with a hand blender. Cook it until it starts boiling and reduce its heat. Add potato in it and cook it for an additional 20 to 30 minutes and it is ready to serve.

Nutrition:

Carbohydrates 51g, protein 17g, fats 6g, calories 310.

Chapter 8: Salads

Cucumber Edamame Salad

Preparation time: 5 minutes
Cooking time: 8 minutes
Servings: 2

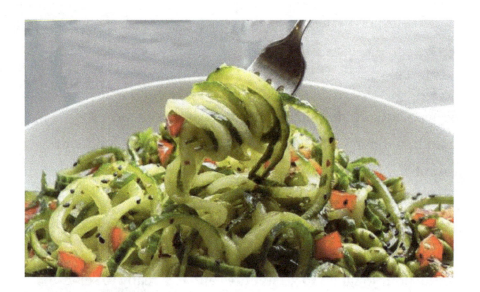

Ingredients:

- 3 tbsp. Avocado oil
- 1 cup cucumber, sliced into thin rounds
- ½ cup fresh sugar snap peas, sliced or whole
- ½ cup fresh edamame
- ¼ cup radish, sliced
- 1 large avocado, peeled, pitted, sliced

- 1 nori sheet, crumbled
- 2 tsp. Roasted sesame seeds
- 1 tsp. Salt

Directions:
Bring a medium-sized pot filled halfway with water to a boil over medium-high heat.
Add the sugar snaps and cook them for about 2 minutes.
Take the pot off the heat, drain the excess water, transfer the sugar snaps to a medium-sized bowl and set aside for now.
Fill the pot with water again, add the teaspoon of salt and bring to a boil over medium-high heat.
Add the edamame to the pot and let them cook for about 6 minutes.
Take the pot off the heat, drain the excess water, transfer the soybeans to the bowl with sugar snaps and let them cool down for about 5 minutes.
Combine all ingredients, except the nori crumbs and roasted sesame seeds, in a medium-sized bowl.
Carefully stir, using a spoon, until all ingredients are evenly coated in oil.
Top the salad with the nori crumbs and roasted sesame seeds.
Transfer the bowl to the fridge and allow the salad to cool for at least 30 minutes.
Nutrition: Calories 409; Carbohydrates 7.1 g; Fats 38.25g; Protein 7.6 g

Best Broccoli Salad

Preparation time: 15 minutes | chilling time: 1 hour | servings: 8

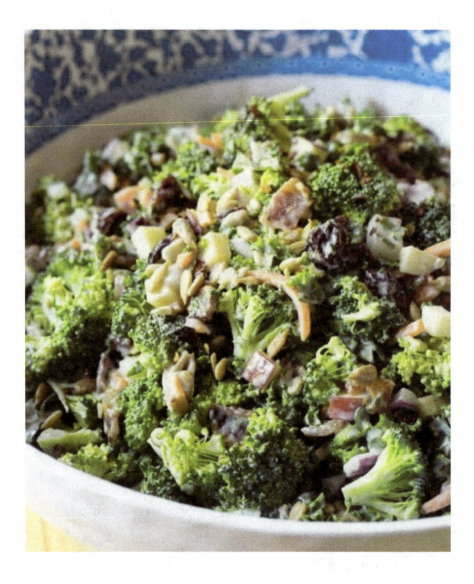

Ingredients:

- 8 cups diced broccoli
- ¼ cup sunflower seeds
- 3 tablespoons apple cider vinegar
- ½ cup dried cranberries
- 1/3 cup cubed onion
- 1 cup mayonnaise
- ½ cup bacon bits
- 2 tablespoons sugar
- ½ teaspoon salt and ground black pepper

Directions:

In a bowl, mix vinegar, salt, pepper, mayonnaise, and sugar. Mix it well. In another bowl, mix all the remaining ingredients and pour the prepared mayonnaise dressing and mix it well. Before serving to refrigerate it for at least an hour.

Nutrition:

Carbohydrates 17g, protein 6g, fats 26g, calories 317

Rainbow Orzo Salad

Preparation time: 10 minutes
Cooking time: 20 minutes
Servings: 1

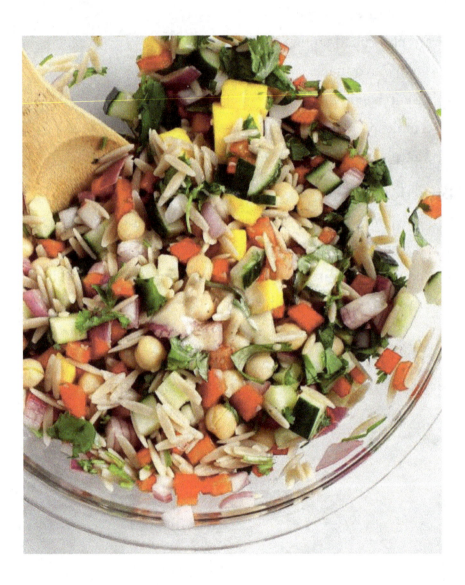

Ingredients:

- 1 chopped onion
- 25g grated feta cheese
- 2 sliced bell peppers
- 1 tablespoon olive oil
- 6 sliced tomatoes
- 2 tablespoons chopped basil
- 25g orzo pasta

Directions:

Preheat the oven at 350f temperature. Prepare a baking sheet and place the onion and bell peppers and drizzle half olive oil. Bake it for around 15 minutes. Add tomatoes on it and bake for an additional 5 minutes. Meanwhile, cook the orzo according to the given directions on the pack and cool it. Now toss it with the baked vegetables and top it with cheese, basil and remaining oil and serve it.

Nutrition:

Carbohydrates 52g, protein 13g, fats 18g, calories 422, sugar 30g.

Broccoli Pasta Salad

Preparation time: 15 minutes
Chilling time: 30 minutes
Servings: 12

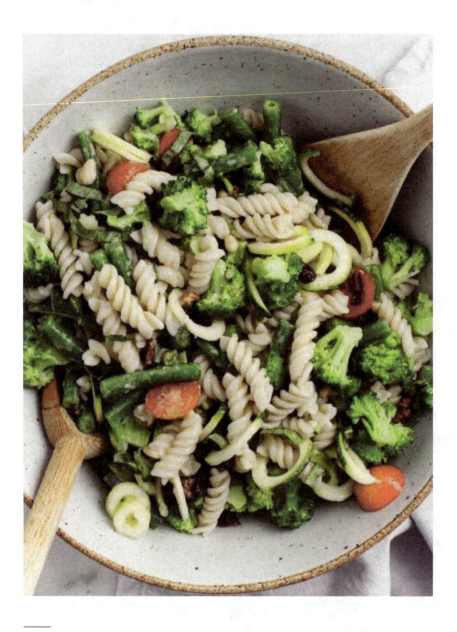

Ingredients:
- 1-pound cooked pasta
- 2 diced broccoli florets
- 1 chopped onion
- 1 cup grated cheese
- 12 ounce cooked and finely chopped bacon
- ¾ teaspoon salt
- ¾ teaspoon ground black pepper
- 1 cup mayonnaise

Directions:
Take a bowl and mix all the ingredients until all of them combined well. Cover it with the plastic wrap and place it in the refrigerator for at least 30 minutes and serve it. You can keep it in the refrigerator for 3 days.

Nutrition:
Carbohydrates 36g, protein 14g, fats 29g, calories 461.

Eggplant & Roasted Tomato Farro Salad

Preparation time: 1 hour
Cooking time: 1 hour 30 minutes
Servings: 3

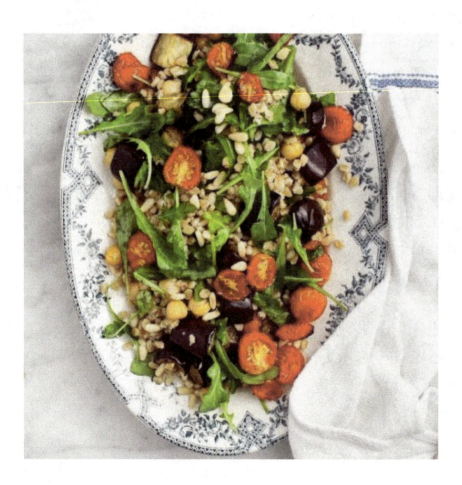

Ingredients:

- 4 small eggplants
- 1 ½ cups chopped cherry tomatoes
- ¾ cup uncooked faro

- 1 tablespoon olive oil
- 1 minced garlic clove
- ½ cup rinsed and drained chickpeas
- 1 tablespoon basil
- 1 tablespoon arugula
- ½ teaspoon salt and ground black pepper
- 1 tablespoon vinegar
- ½ cup toasted pine nuts

Directions:

Preheat the oven at 300f temperature and prepare a baking sheet. Place cherry tomatoes on the baking liner and drizzle olive oil, salt, and black pepper on it and bake it for 30 to 35 minutes. Cook the faro in the salted water for 30 to 40 minutes. Slice the eggplant and salt it and leave it for 30 minutes. After that, rinse it with water and dry it kitchen towel. Now peeled and sliced the eggplants. Now place these slices on the baking liner and season it with salt, pepper and olive oil. Bake it for 15 to 20 minutes in the preheated oven at the 450f temperature. Flip the sides of eggplant and bake it for an additional 15 to 20 minutes. Bake the pine nuts for 5 minutes and sauté the garlic. Now mix all the ingredients in a bowl and serve it.

Nutrition:

Carbohydrates 37g, protein 9g, fats 25g, calories 399.

Summer Corn Salad

Preparation time: 5 minutes
Servings: 8

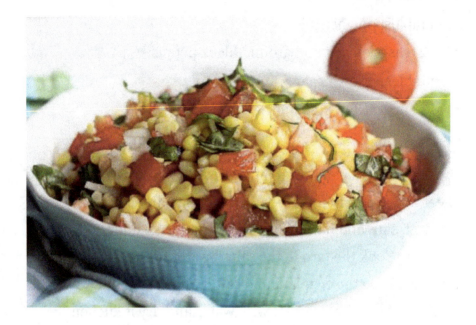

Ingredients:

- 4 ears corn
- 1 diced red bell pepper
- 1 cubed green bell pepper
- 1 cubed onion
- 2 tablespoons olive oil
- 1 tablespoon lemon juice
- ½ cup chopped fresh cilantro
- ½ teaspoon salt and ground black pepper

Directions:

Shave the corns off from the cob. Take a bowl and mix all the ingredients until all the ingredients combined well and it is ready to serve.

Nutrition:

Carbohydrates 16g, protein 4g, fats 8g, calories 136

Best Tomato and Avocado Salad

Preparation time: 5 minutes
Servings: 4

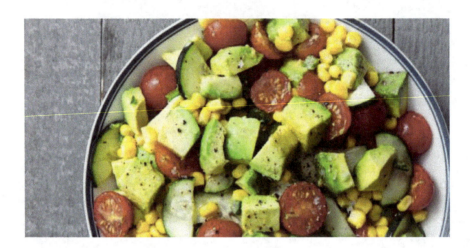

Ingredients:

- 2 cups sliced tomatoes
- ¼ sliced onion
- 1 tablespoon lemon juice
- 2 cubed avocados
- ¼ cup chopped parsley
- ½ teaspoon red pepper flakes
- 2 tablespoons olive oil
- ½ teaspoon salt and ground black pepper

Directions:

Add tomatoes, cilantro, and avocado in a salad bowl. Now add remaining ingredients in it and mix it well. Now it is ready to serve. It is up to you. Whether you serve it immediately or serve it after refrigerating it.

Nutrition:

Carbohydrates 12g, protein 2g, fats 19g, calories 214, sugar 4g.

Sweet Pepper Panzanella

Preparation time: 15 minutes
Servings: 4

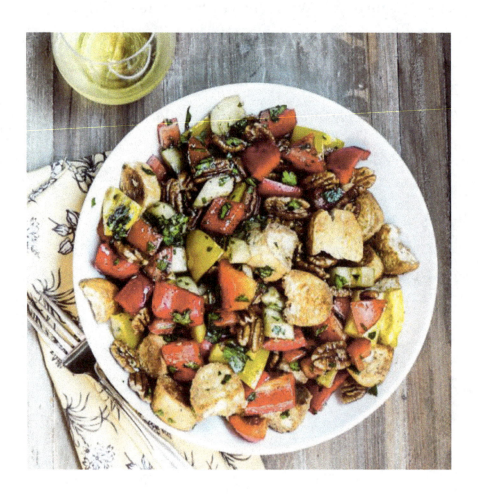

Ingredients:

- 2 lb. Red or orange bell peppers
- ½ thinly sliced onion
- 2 minced garlic cloves

- 8 tablespoons olive oil
- 2 tablespoons vinegar
- 2 minced garlic cloves
- 2 tablespoons fresh oregano
- ½ teaspoon salt and ground black pepper
- ¼ teaspoon crushed red pepper flakes
- 4 ounces fresh mozzarella
- ½ crushed loaf bread
- ¼ cup fresh mint leaves

Directions:

Preheat the boiler and toss the bell peppers with olive oil, salt, and black pepper. Cook it for around 10 to 12 minutes. In a large bowl, add peppers, onion, garlic, vinegar, red pepper flakes. Olive oil and mix it well. Now bake the bread and season it with remaining oil, salt, and pepper. Bake it for around 8 to 10 minutes in the preheated oven at the 400f temperature. Now mix all the baked and raw materials and mix them well.

Nutrition:

Carbohydrates 37g, protein 17g, fats 15g, calories 426, sugar 4g.

Purple Potato and Green Bean Salad

Preparation time: 15 minutes
Cooking time: 15 minutes
Servings: 8

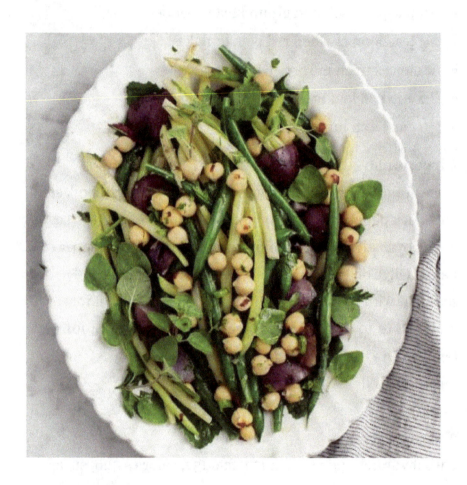

Ingredients:

- 2 pounds diced potatoes
- ½ cup chopped celery
- 2 cups fresh green beans

- 1 tablespoon salt
- ¾ cup mayonnaise
- ½ cup chopped onion
- 2 tablespoons lime juice
- 2 teaspoons chopped the dill
- ¾ cup mayonnaise
- 2 tablespoons sour cream
- ½ teaspoon ground black pepper

Directions:

Put the potatoes in the saucepan and cover it with salty water. Cook it for around 15 minutes. Boil the beans for around 5 to 7 minutes. In a bowl, add all the ingredients and merge them well and it is ready to serve.

Nutrition:

Carbohydrates 51g, protein 7g, fats 15g, calories 307

Spinach and Mashed Tofu Salad

Preparation time: 20 minutes

Servings: 4

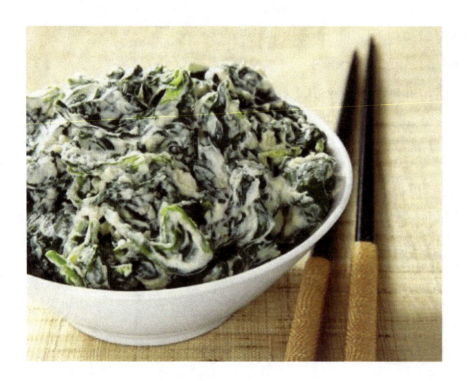

Ingredients:

- 2 8-oz. Blocks firm tofu, drained
- 4 cups baby spinach leaves
- 4 tbsp. Cashew butter
- 1½ tbsp. Soy sauce
- 1-inch piece ginger, finely chopped
- 1 tsp. Red miso paste
- 2 tbsp. Sesame seeds

- 1 tsp. Organic orange zest
- 1 tsp. Nori flakes
- 2 tbsp. Water

Directions:

Use paper towels to absorb any excess water left in the tofu before crumbling both blocks into small pieces.

In a large bowl, combine the mashed tofu with the spinach leaves.

Mix the remaining ingredients in another small bowl and, if desired, add the optional water for a smoother dressing.

Pour this dressing over the mashed tofu and spinach leaves. Transfer the bowl to the fridge and allow the salad to chill for up to one hour. Doing so will guarantee a better flavor. Or, the salad can be served right away.

Nutrition:

Calories 166

Carbohydrates 5.5 g

Fats 10.7 g

Protein 11.3 g

Chapter 9: Side Dishes

Garden Patch Sandwiches on Multigrain Bread

Preparation time: 15 minutes
Cooking time: 0 minutes
Servings: 4 sandwiches

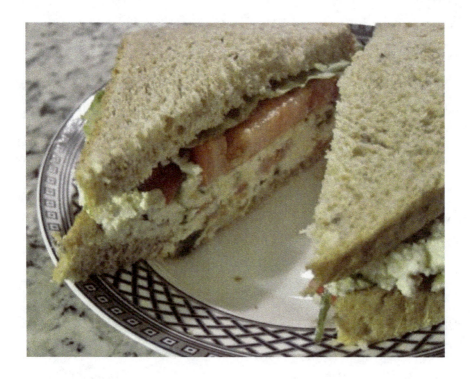

Ingredients:
- 1pound extra-firm tofu, drained and patted dry
- 1 medium red bell pepper, finely chopped
- 1 celery rib, finely chopped

- 3 green onions, minced
- 1/4 cup shelled sunflower seeds
- 1/2 cup vegan mayonnaise, homemade or store-bought
- 1/2 teaspoon salt
- 1/2 teaspoon celery salt
- 1/4 teaspoon freshly ground black pepper
- 8 slices whole grain bread
- 4 (1/4-inch) slices ripe tomato
- 4 lettuce leaves

Directions:

Crumble the tofu and place it in a large bowl. Add the bell pepper, celery, green onions, and sunflower seeds. Stir in the mayonnaise, salt, celery salt, and pepper and mix until well combined.

Toast the bread, if desired. Spread the mixture evenly onto 4 slices of the bread. Top each with a tomato slice, lettuce leaf, and the remaining bread. Cut the sandwiches diagonally in half and serve.

Garden Salad Wraps

Preparation time: 15 minutes
Cooking time: 10 minutes
Servings: 4 wraps

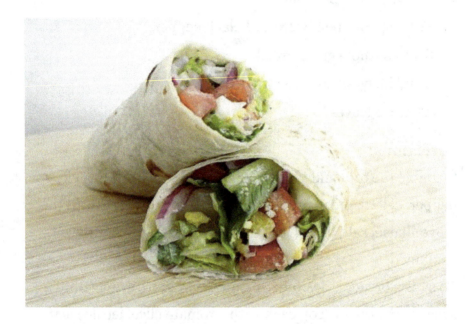

Ingredients:
- 6 tablespoons olive oil
- 1-pound extra-firm tofu, drained, patted dry, and cut into ½-inch strips
- 1 tablespoon soy sauce
- ¼ cup apple cider vinegar
- 1 teaspoon yellow or spicy brown mustard
- ½ teaspoon salt
- ¼ teaspoon freshly ground black pepper

- 3 cups shredded romaine lettuce
- 3 ripe roma tomatoes, finely chopped
- 1 large carrot, shredded
- 1 medium english cucumber, peeled and chopped
- 1/3 cup minced red onion
- 1/4 cup sliced pitted green olives
- 4 (10-inch) whole-grain flour tortillas or lavash flatbread

Directions:

In a large skillet, heat 2 tablespoons of the oil over medium heat. Add the tofu and cook until golden brown, about 10 minutes. Sprinkle with soy sauce and set aside to cool.

In a small bowl, combine the vinegar, mustard, salt, and pepper with the remaining 4 tablespoons oil, stirring to blend well. Set aside.

In a large bowl, combine the lettuce, tomatoes, carrot, cucumber, onion, and olives. Pour on the dressing and toss to coat.

To assemble wraps, place 1 tortilla on a work surface and spread with about one-quarter of the salad. Place a few strips of tofu on the tortilla and roll up tightly. Slice in half

Marinated Mushroom Wraps

Preparation time: 15 minutes
Cooking time: 0 minutes
Servings: 2 wraps

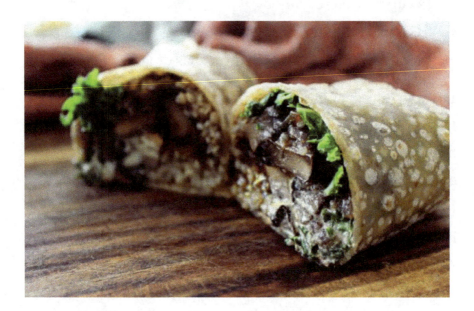

Ingredients:

- 3 tablespoons soy sauce
- 3 tablespoons fresh lemon juice
- 1½ tablespoons toasted sesame oil
- 2 portobello mushroom caps, cut into ¼-inch strips
- 1 ripe hass avocado, pitted and peeled
- 2 cups fresh baby spinach leaves
- 1 medium red bell pepper, cut into ¼-inch strips
- 1 ripe tomato, chopped

- Salt and freshly ground black pepper

Directions:

In a medium bowl, combine the soy sauce, 2 tablespoons of the lemon juice, and the oil. Add the portobello strips, toss to combine, and marinate for 1 hour or overnight. Drain the mushrooms and set aside.

Mash the avocado with the remaining 1 tablespoon of lemon juice.

To assemble wraps, place 1 tortilla on a work surface and spread with some of the mashed avocado. Top with a layer of baby spinach leaves. In the lower third of each tortilla, arrange strips of the soaked mushrooms and some of the bell pepper strips. Sprinkle with the tomato and salt and black pepper to taste. Roll up tightly and cut in half diagonally. Repeat with the remaining ingredients and serve.

Tamari Toasted Almonds

Preparation time: 2 minutes
Cooking time: 8 minutes
Servings: ½ cup

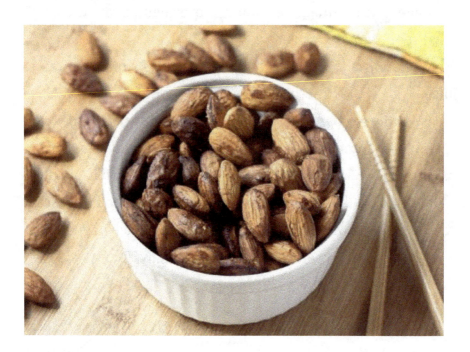

Ingredients:

- ½ cup raw almonds, or sunflower seeds
- 2 tablespoons tamari, or soy sauce
- 1 teaspoon toasted sesame oil

Directions:
Preparing the ingredients.

Heat a dry skillet to medium-high heat, then add the almonds, stirring very frequently to keep them from burning. Once the almonds are toasted, 7 to 8 minutes for almonds, or 3 to 4 minutes for sunflower seeds, pour the tamari and sesame oil into the hot skillet and stir to coat.

You can turn off the heat, and as the almonds cool the tamari mixture will stick to and dry on the nuts.

Per serving (1 tablespoon) calories: 89; total fat: 8g; carbs: 3g; fiber: 2g; protein: 4g

Avocado and Tempeh Bacon Wraps

Preparation time: 10 minutes
Cooking time: 8 minutes
Servings: 4 wraps

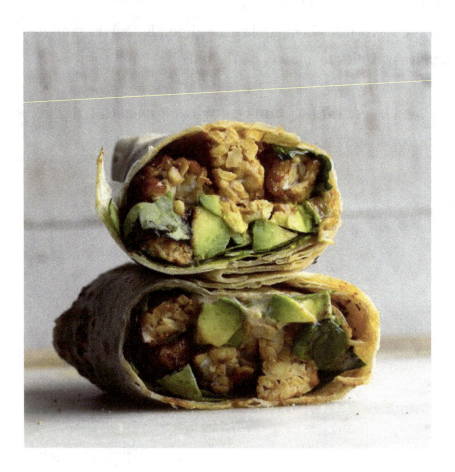

Ingredients:

- 2 tablespoons olive oil
- 8 ounces tempeh bacon, homemade or store-bought
- 4 (10-inch) soft flour tortillas or lavash flat bread

- 1/4 cup vegan mayonnaise, homemade or store-bought
- 4 large lettuce leaves
- 2 ripe hass avocados, pitted, peeled, and cut into 1/4-inch slices
- 1 large ripe tomato, cut into 1/4-inch slices

Directions:

In a large skillet, heat the oil over medium heat. Add the tempeh bacon and cook until browned on both sides, about 8 minutes. Remove from the heat and set aside.

Place 1 tortilla on a work surface. Spread with some of the mayonnaise and one-fourth of the lettuce and tomatoes.

Pit, peel, and thinly slice the avocado and place the slices on top of the tomato. Add the reserved tempeh bacon and roll up tightly. Repeat with remaining ingredients and serve.

Stuffed Cherry Tomatoes

Preparation time: 15 minutes
Cooking time: 0 minutes
Servings: 6

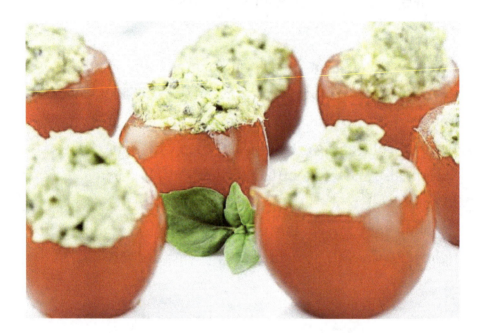

Ingredients:

- 2 pints cherry tomatoes, tops removed and centers scooped out
- 2 avocados, mashed
- Juice of 1 lemon
- ½ red bell pepper, minced
- 4 green onions (white and green parts), finely minced
- 1 tablespoon minced fresh tarragon

- Pinch of sea salt

Directions:

Preparing the ingredients.

Place the cherry tomatoes open-side up on a platter.

In a small bowl, -combine the avocado, lemon juice, bell pepper, scallions, tarragon, and salt.

Stir until well -combined. Scoop into the cherry tomatoes and serve immediately.

Spicy Black Bean Dip

Preparation time: 10 minutes
Cooking time: 0 minutes
Servings: 2 cups

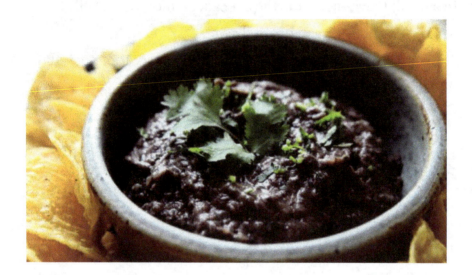

Ingredients:

- 1 (14-ounce) can black beans, drained and rinsed, or 1½ cups cooked
- Zest and juice of 1 lime
- 1 tablespoon tamari, or soy sauce
- ¼ cup water
- ¼ cup fresh cilantro, chopped
- 1 teaspoon ground cumin
- Pinch cayenne pepper

Directions:

Preparing the ingredients.

Put the beans in a food processor (best choice) or blender, along with the lime zest and juice, tamari, and about ¼ cup of water.

Blend until smooth, then blend in the cilantro, cumin, and cayenne.

If you don't have a blender or prefer a different consistency, simply transfer it to a bowl once the beans have been puréed and stir in the spices, instead of forcing the blender.

Per serving (1 cup) calories: 190; total fat: 1g; carbs: 35g; fiber: 12g; protein: 13g

French Onion Pastry Puffs

Preparation time: 10 minutes
Cooking time: 35 minutes - makes 24 puffs

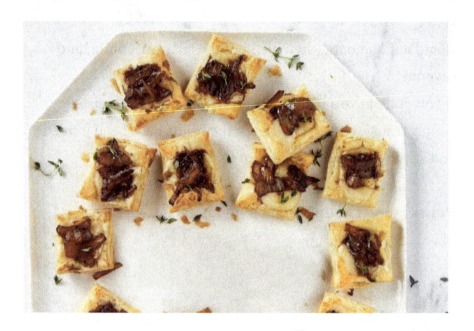

Ingredients:

- 1 tablespoon capers
- 1 sheet frozen vegan puff pastry, thawed
- 18 pitted black olives, quartered

Directions:

In a medium skillet, heat the oil over medium heat. Add the onions and garlic, season with rosemary and salt and pepper to taste. Cover and cook until very soft, stirring occasionally, about 20 minutes. Stir in the capers and set aside.

Preheat the oven to 400°f. Roll out the puff pastry and cut into 2-to 3-inch circles using a lightly floured pastry cutter or drinking glass. You should get about 2 dozen circles.

Arrange the pastry circles on baking sheets and top each with a heaping teaspoon of onion mixture, patting down to smooth the top.

Top with 3 olive quarters, arranged decoratively—either like flower petals emanating from the center or parallel to each other like 3 bars.

Bake until pastry is puffed and golden brown, about 15 minutes. Serve hot.

Salsa Fresca

Preparation time: 15 minutes
Cooking time: 0 minutes
Servings: 4

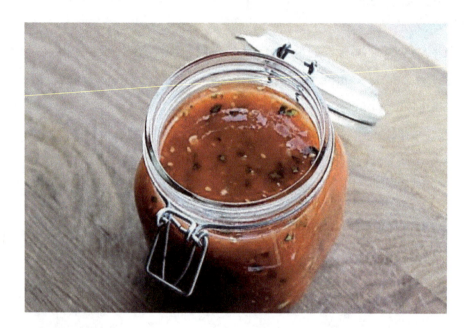

Ingredients:

- 3 large heirloom tomatoes or other fresh tomatoes, chopped
- ½ red onion, finely chopped
- ½ bunch cilantro, chopped
- 2 garlic cloves, minced
- 1 jalapeño, minced
- Juice of 1 lime, or 1 tablespoon prepared lime juice
- ¼ cup olive oil

- Sea salt
- Whole-grain tortilla chips, for serving

Directions:

Preparing the ingredients.

In a small bowl, combine the tomatoes, onion, cilantro, garlic, jalapeño, lime juice, and olive oil and mix well. Allow to sit at room temperature for 15 minutes. Season with salt.

Serve with tortilla chips.

The salsa can be stored in an airtight container in the refrigerator for up to 1 week.

Lemon and Garlic Marinated Mushrooms

Preparation time: 15 minutes
Cooking time: 0 minutes
Servings: 4 servings

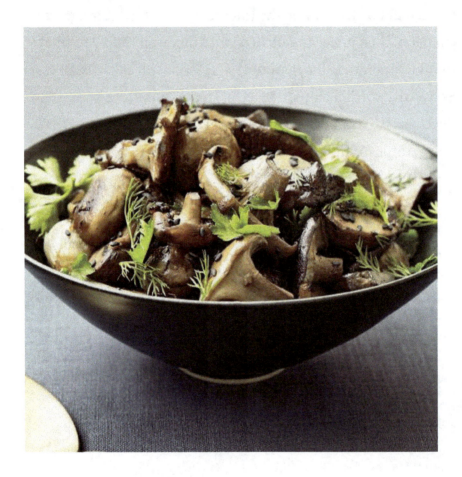

Ingredients:

- 3 tablespoons olive oil
- 2 tablespoons fresh lemon juice
- 2 garlic cloves, crushed

- 1 teaspoon dried marjoram
- ½ teaspoon coarsely ground fennel seed
- ½ teaspoon salt
- ¼ teaspoon freshly ground black pepper
- 8 ounces small white mushrooms, lightly rinsed, patted dry, and stemmed
- 1 tablespoon minced fresh parsley

Directions:

In a medium bowl, whisk together the oil, lemon juice, garlic, marjoram, fennel seed, salt, and pepper. Add the mushrooms and parsley and stir gently until coated.

Cover and refrigerate for at least 2 hours or overnight. Stir well before serving.

Garlic Toast

Preparation time: 5 minutes
Cooking time: 5 minutes
Servings: 1 slice

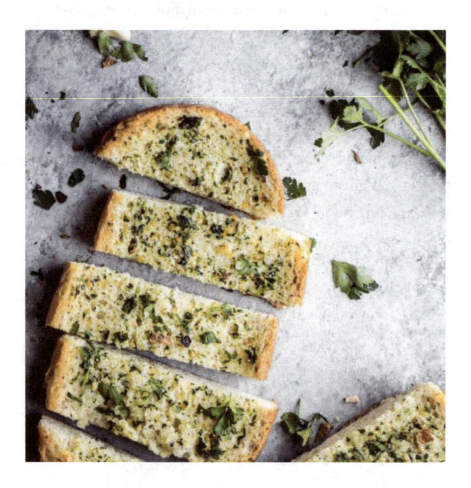

Ingredients:

- 1 teaspoon coconut oil, or olive oil
- Pinch sea salt
- 1 to 2 teaspoons nutritional yeast

- 1 small garlic clove, pressed, or ¼ teaspoon garlic powder
- 1 slice whole-grain bread

Directions:

Preparing the ingredients.

In a small bowl, mix together the oil, salt, nutritional yeast, and garlic.

You can either toast the bread and then spread it with the seasoned oil, or brush the oil on the bread and put it in a toaster oven to bake for 5 minutes.

If you're using fresh garlic, it's best to spread it onto the bread and then bake it.

Per serving (1 slice) calories: 138; total fat: 6g; carbs: 16g; fiber: 4g; protein: 7g

Vietnamese-Style Lettuce Rolls

Preparation time: 15 minutes
Cooking time: 0 minutes
Servings: 4 servings

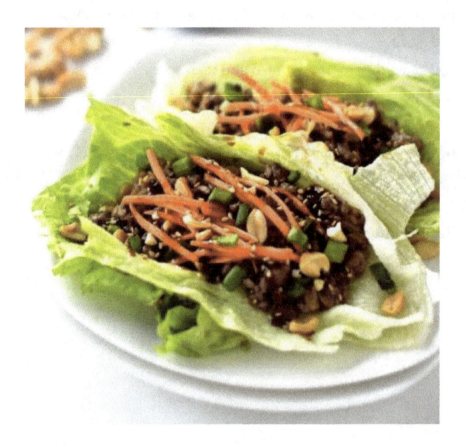

Ingredients:

- 2 green onions
- 2 tablespoons soy sauce
- 2 tablespoons rice vinegar
- 1 teaspoon sugar

- 1/8 teaspoon crushed red pepper
- 3 tablespoons water
- 3 ounces rice vermicelli
- 4 to 6 soft green leaf lettuce leaves
- 1 medium carrot, shredded
- 1/2 medium english cucumber, peeled, seeded, and cut lengthwise into 1/4-inch strips
- 1/2 medium red bell pepper, cut into 1/4-inch strips
- 1 cup loosely packed fresh cilantro or basil leaves

Directions:

Cut the green part off the green onions and cut them lengthwise into thin slices and set aside. Mince the white part of the green onions and transfer to a small bowl. Add the soy sauce, rice vinegar, sugar, crushed red pepper, and water. Stir to blend and set aside.

Soak the vermicelli in medium bowl of hot water until softened, about 1 minute. Drain the noodles well and cut them into 3-inch lengths. Set aside.

Place a lettuce leaf on a work surface and arrange a row of noodles in the center of the leaf, followed by a few strips of scallion greens, carrot, cucumber, bell pepper, and cilantro. Bring the bottom edge of the leaf over the filling and fold in the two short sides. Roll up gently but tightly. Place the roll seam side down on a serving platter. Repeat with Remaining ingredients. Serve with the dipping sauce.

Chapter 10: Pasta and Noodles

Pasta with Roasted Red Pepper Sauce

Preparation time: 10 minutes
Cooking time: 10 minutes
Servings: 6

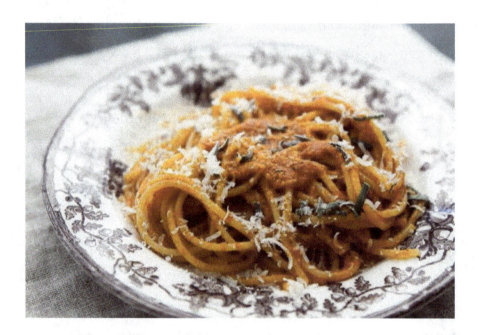

Ingredients:

- 1-pound cooked pasta
- 2 tablespoons butter
- ½ diced onion
- 1 tablespoon olive oil
- 3 minced garlic cloves

- 1 cup vegetable broth
- 16 ounces roasted red pepper
- 2 tablespoons minced fresh parsley
- ¼ cup cream
- ½ cup chopped fresh basil
- ½ cup shredded parmesan

Directions:

In a skillet, add butter and oil and cook it over medium flame. Add onion and garlic in it and cook it for 2 to 3 minutes. Stir red peppers in it and cook for 3 minutes. Now blend the prepared batter and blend it well. Pour the blended puree in the skillet and add broth, salt, and black pepper in it and stir it well. Add basil and parsley in it and combine all the ingredients well. Now add pasta and cheese in it and mix it well. It is ready to serve.

Nutrition:

Carbohydrates 75g, protein 14g, fats 14g, calories 487, sugar 4g

Macaroni and Cheese

Preparation time: 10 minutes
Cooking time: 15 minutes
Servings: 9

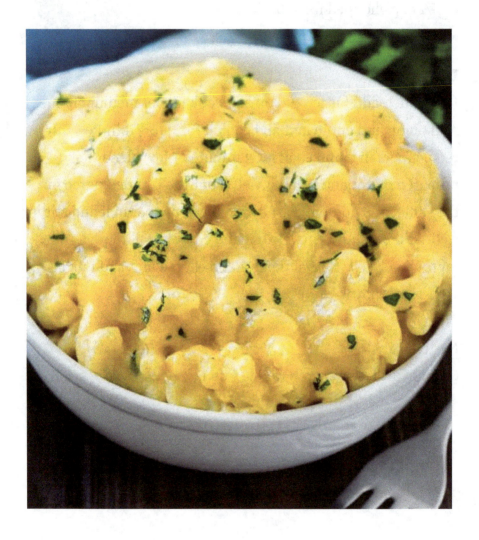

Ingredients:

- 14 oz. Macaroni
- 2 1/3 cups low fat milk
- 3 ½ tablespoons flour
- ¼ teaspoon garlic powder
- 3 ½ tablespoons butter
- ½ teaspoon salt
- ½ teaspoon dry mustard
- 8 oz. Grated cheddar cheese
- 4 oz. Diced cream cheese
- 4 oz. Grated mozzarella cheese
- ½ cup reserved boiled pasta water

Directions:

Take a big pan with water to boil the pasta. Boil the pasta according to the given directions. Drain pasta and reserve some water. Take a pand melt the butter over medium flame and add flour in it. Cook it for around one minute and whisk it continuously. While cooking it, gradually pour milk in it and add garlic powder, and mustard in it and mix it well and increase the heat gradually. Now reduce the heat and add cream cheese in it and mix it until it melted. Remove the pan from the stove and add cheese and season it with salt. Now mix all the ingredients and serve it immediately.

Nutrition:

Carbohydrates 39g, protein 9g, fats 21g, calories 427, sugar 4g

Veggies Soba Noodles with Marinated Tofu

Preparation time: 15 minutes
Cooking time: 20 minutes
Servings: 8

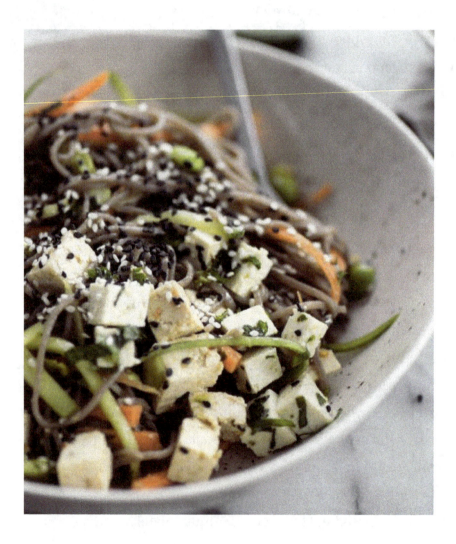

Ingredients:

- 1 teaspoon grated ginger
- 2 tablespoons olive oil
- 8 ounces pressed and drained tofu
- ¼ cup chopped mint
- ¼ cup chopped cilantro
- 8 ounces soba noodles
- 1 diced carrot
- 2 peeled and diced cucumbers
- 2 chopped scallions
- ¾ cup edamame
- 2 tablespoons black sesame seeds

Directions:

In a bowl, whisk ginger, olive oil, mint, and cilantro. Now marinate the tofu in this mixture for around 30 minutes. Take a large pot with water to boil the soba noodles. Boil the noodles according to the given directions, remove the boiling water, rinse it with cold water, and set aside. Now take a bowl, add all the ingredients, and whisk them well until all the ingredients merged well. It is suggested to serve it after an hour or at least after 20 to 30 minutes.

Nutrition:

Carbohydrates 113g, protein 34g, fats 22g, calories 775

Cambodian Vegetable Stir-Fry

Preparation time: 15 minutes
Cooking time: 30 minutes
Servings: 8

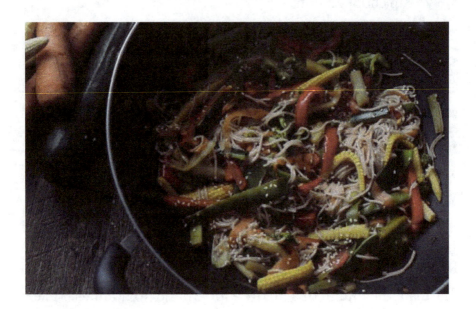

Ingredients:

- 4 diced onions
- 4 stripped cut corns
- ½ pack brown rice vermicelli noodles
- 2 drops sesame oil
- 1 minced garlic clove
- 1 tablespoon grapeseed oil
- 1 cubed carrot
- ½ diced capsicum

- ¼ cup sliced snow peas
- 1 sliced zucchini
- ½ diced broccoli florets
- 1 chopped red chili
- 2 tablespoons tamari
- ¼ cup pineapple puree
- ¼ cup of water
- 2 tablespoons coconut sugar
- ½ teaspoon salt

Directions:

Cook the noodles by following the directions given on the pack. In a pan heat, the sesame oil and grapeseed oil and add garlic in it and cook all the vegetables. Now take the salt, tamari, pineapple puree, sugar, and water and mix all these ingredients well to make the sauce. When vegetables are cooked, add the prepared sauce in it, cool it for an additional 2 minutes, add cooked noodles in it, and cook. Now it is ready to serve.

Nutrition:

Carbohydrates 20.4g, protein 20.3g, fats 7.9g, calories 234

Roasted Garlic Tomato Spaghetti with Garlic Parmesan Bread Crumbs

Preparation time: 10 minutes
Cooking time: 30 minutes
Servings: 3

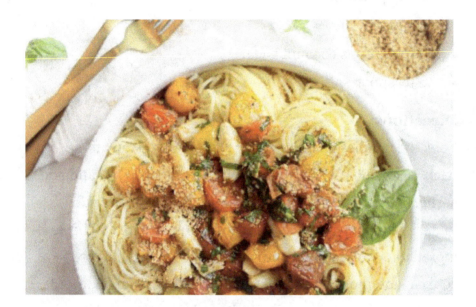

Ingredients:

- 8 ounces spaghetti
- 12 ounces sliced cherry tomatoes
- 1/8 cup vegan parmesan
- ¼ teaspoon garlic powder
- 1/8 cup bread crumbs
- ½ cup olive oil
- 1 minced garlic

- ¼ cup chopped fresh basil
- 1 tablespoon chopped rosemary
- ½ teaspoon salt and ground black pepper

Directions:

In a skillet, add ½-teaspoon olive oil, cook parmesan, breadcrumbs, and garlic powder, and cook it over medium flame. Stir it continuously and when its color changed to brown, remove it from the stove. Preheat the oven at 400f temperature. Prepare a baking dish with a baking line. Now place tomatoes, garlic, and rosemary and season it with salt, black pepper, and olive oil. Moreover, bake it for around 10 to 12 minutes. Prepare spaghetti and boil it for around 8 to 10 minutes according to the instructed time. Reserve one cup of spaghetti water and drain the remaining water. Now place the pasta back on the stove over a low flame and add remaining olive oil, baked tomatoes, basil and cooked garlic mixture in it and the reserved pasta water. Cook it for 5 to 6 minutes until sauce reaches the required consistency. Serve it with toasted breadcrumbs.

Nutrition:

Carbohydrates 53g, protein 20g, fats 18g, calories 450

Zoodle Pad Thai

Preparation time: 10 minutes
Cooking time: 15 minutes
Servings: 2

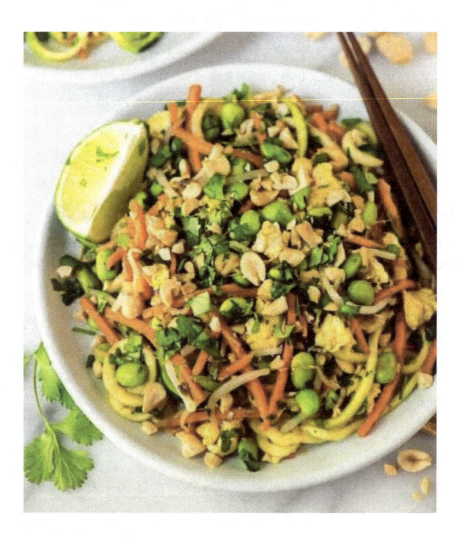

Ingredients:

- 2 eggs

- 1 minced garlic clove
- ½ tablespoon olive oil
- 1 tablespoon coconut flour
- ¼ cup roasted ground peanuts
- 1 minced shallot
- 2 sliced zucchini
- 1 tablespoon chopped cilantro
- ½ tablespoon soy sauce
- 2 tablespoons lemon juice
- 1 tablespoon chili sauce
- 1 tablespoon fish sauce
- 1 teaspoon honey

Directions:

In a bowl, add honey, fish sauce, lemon juice, chili sauce, and soy sauce and stir it well. Scramble the eggs and put it aside. On the medium flame, place a skillet and add oil, shallots, and garlic and cook it for about 2 minutes. Now pour the prepared sauce in it and stir it. Now add coconut flour in it and whisk it quickly, so the sauce gets thicker. Put zucchini noodles and chopped cilantro in it and combine it thoroughly. Cook it for an additional 2 minutes and add scrambled eggs and ground peanut in it and cook for around 1 minute and serve it.

Nutrition:

Carbohydrates 186g, protein 15g, fats 17g, calories 308, sugar 18g.

Peanut Vegetable Noodle Bowl

Preparation time: 10 minutes
Cooking time: 10 minutes
Servings: 4

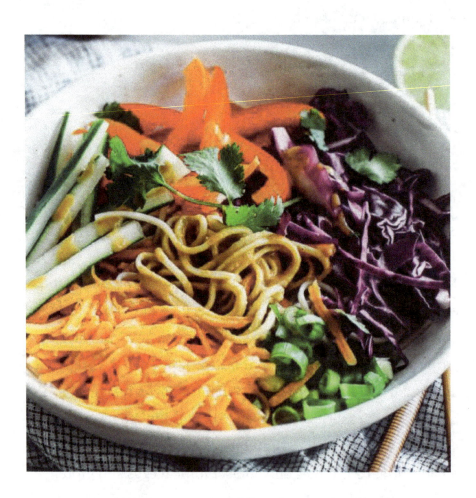

Ingredients:

- ½ cup thinly sliced bell pepper
- 8 oz. Noodles

- 1 thin sliced carrot
- ½ thin sliced cucumber
- ½ cup chopped cilantro
- 1/3 cup chopped peanuts
- 1 chopped onion
- 2 tablespoons toasted sesame oil
- ¼ cup peanut butter
- 2 tablespoons pure maple syrup
- 1 tablespoon minced garlic and ginger
- 1 tablespoon apple cider vinegar

Directions:

Cook the noodles by following the directions given on the package. After cooking it, drain the water and rinse it with cold water and put it aside. In a bowl, add peanut butter, sesame oil, vinegar, ginger, garlic, maples syrup, and soy sauce and combine it well. In another bowl, add noodles and add all the remaining ingredients in it and serve it.

Nutrition:

Carbohydrates 74g, protein 12g, fats 24g, calories 553, sugar 22g.

Garlic Pasta with Roasted Brussels Sprouts And Tomatoes

Preparation time: 15 minutes
Cooking time: 45 minutes
Servings: 8

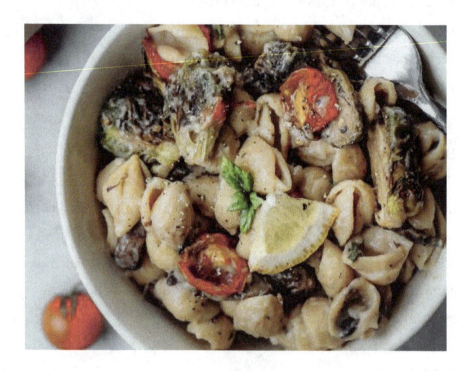

Ingredients:

- 1 cup halved Brussel sprout
- 1 teaspoon olive oil
- 2 minced garlic cloves
- ½ cup sliced cherry tomatoes
- 1 cup sliced mushrooms

- ¼ cubed onion
- 2 cups almond milk
- ¼ cup flour
- 2 teaspoons lemon juice
- ½ teaspoon lemon zest
- ½ teaspoon ground black pepper
- 4 cups pasta
- 1 tablespoon chopped basil
- ½ teaspoon salt

Directions:

Preheat the oven at 400f temperature. Prepare a baking dish with a greased baking sheet. Place Brussel sprout, tomatoes, and garlic cloves in the baking dish and season it with oil, salt, and pepper. Bake it for 30 minutes. Boil the pasta according to the package directions and drain it and set aside. In a skillet with olive oil, cool anion and garlic over the medium flame for about 3 minutes. Add flour and milk in it gradually and stir it continuously. When it combined properly, reduce the heat and cool it for 8 to 10 minutes until the sauce becomes thick. Now add lemon juice, lemon zest, basil, salt, and black pepper in it and cook it for an additional 4 minutes. Add cooked pasta and backed veggies in the sauce and toss it to coat and it is ready to serve.

Nutrition:

Carbohydrates 16g, protein 7g, fats 6g, calories 135, sugar 4g.

Veggies and Noodle Bowl with Mushrooms

Preparation time: 10 minutes

Cooking time: 20 minutes

Servings: 2

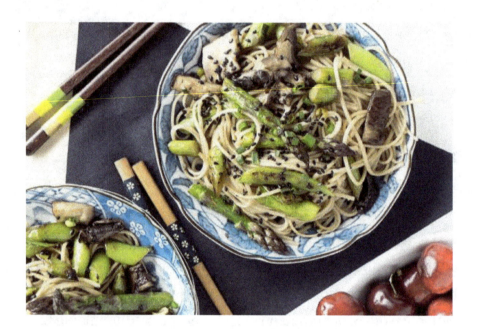

Ingredients:

- 8 ounces sliced mushrooms
- 9 oz. Rinsed and sliced leeks
- 8 ounces noodles
- 5 ounces baby spinach
- 1 tablespoon olive oil
- 3 chopped scallions
- ½ teaspoon salt

- ½ teaspoon black pepper
- 1 tablespoon water
- 1 tablespoon sesame seeds
- 1 tablespoon honey
- 1 tablespoon vinegar
- ¼ cup of soy sauce
- ½ teaspoon ground red pepper flakes
- 1 tablespoon sesame oil

Directions:

In a pan toast the sesame seeds over medium flame for around 5 minutes. Transfer it to a mixing bowl and add vinegar, soy sauce, honey, sesame oil, red pepper, water, and scallion and mix them well. In a pan, add 1 tablespoon oil and heat it over medium flame. Add leeks, mushrooms, scallions, salt, and pepper and cook it for few minutes and remove it from the stove. Cook your noodles according to the given directions and drain them. Now add cooked noodles on a pan with the vegetables and heat it over medium flame and add the sauce in it and cook it until the sauce gets thicker and serve it.

Nutrition:

Carbohydrates 61g, protein 13g, fats 18g, calories 452, sugar 13g.

Veggie Pasta

Preparation time: 15 minutes
Cooking time: 15 minutes
Servings: 8

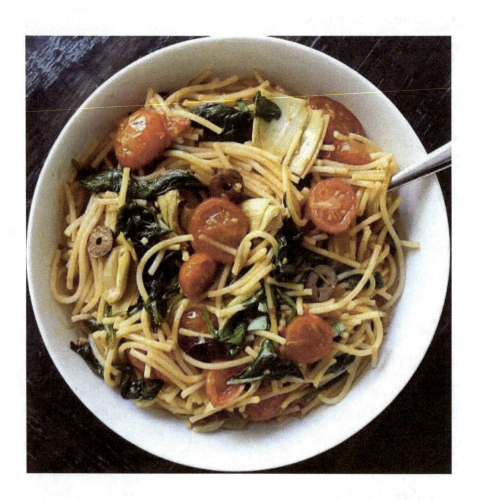

Ingredients:

- 150g pasta
- 2 tablespoons olive oil

- 3 cubed tomatoes
- ½ cup chopped basil
- 150g drained and chopped broccoli
- 1 tablespoon vinegar
- 2 tablespoons chopped chives
- 1 tablespoons baby capers

Directions:

Cook the pasta according to the given directions on the package. In a bowl, add olive oil, vinegar, tomatoes, and capers and mix all the ingredients well. Add the cooked pasta in it and toss it and leave it for around 5 minutes. Now put all the remaining ingredients in it and whisk them well. It is ready to serve.

Nutrition:

Carbohydrates 57g, protein 21g, fats 24g, calories 594, sugar 4.5g

Summer Garlic Scape and Zucchini Pasta

Preparation time: 10 minutes
Cooking time: 10 minutes
Servings: 4

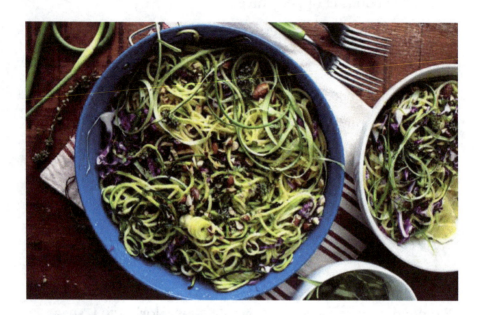

Ingredients:

- 4 zucchinis
- 1 small pack cooked pasta
- ½ thin sliced purple cabbage
- 1 tablespoon olive oil
- 10 minced garlic cloves
- 1 tablespoon lemon juice
- 1 cup lemon thyme
- 2 tablespoons chopped almonds

- ½ teaspoon salt and ground black pepper

Directions:

Preheat the oven at 450f temperature and bake zucchini for around 8 minutes. Take a large bowl, add baked zucchini, cabbage, and pasta in it, and whisk well. Now add all the remaining items in it and mix it and it is ready to serve.

Nutrition:

Carbohydrates 21g, protein 8g, fats 17g, calories 255, sugar 4g

Sun Dried Tomato Pesto Pasta

Preparation time: 15 minutes
Cooking time: 15 minutes
Servings: 5

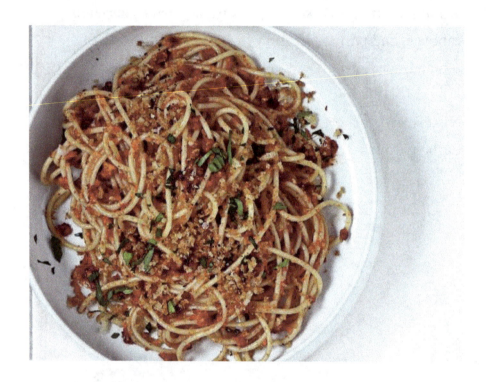

Ingredients:

- 1 cup fresh basil leaves
- 6-ounce sun-dried tomatoes
- 1 tablespoon lemon juice
- ½ teaspoon salt
- ¼ cup olive oil
- ¼ cup almonds

- 3 minced garlic cloves
- ½ teaspoon chopped red pepper flakes
- 8 ounces pasta

Directions:

Cook the pasta according to the given directions. For making, the pesto toasts the almonds over medium flame in a small skillet for around 4 minutes. In a blender, put sun-dried tomatoes, basil, garlic, lemon juice, salt, red pepper flakes, and toasted almonds and blend it. While blending, add olive oil in it and blend it until it converts in the form of pesto. Now coat the pasta with the pesto and serve it.

Nutrition:

Carbohydrates 34g, protein 30g, fats 9g, calories 345, sugar 10g

Zucchini Pasta with Spicy Tomato and Lentil Sauce

Preparation time: 10 minutes
Cooking time: 55 minutes
Servings: 2

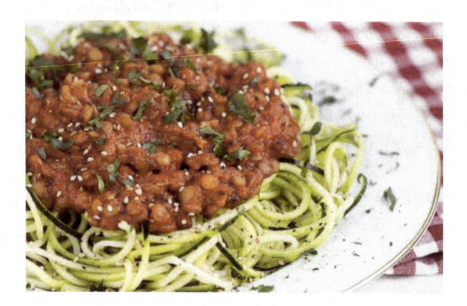

Ingredients:

- ½ cup tomato paste
- 2 minced garlic
- ¾ cup dry green lentils
- 1 cubed onion
- 1 teaspoon vinegar
- 1 ¼ cups of water
- 1 teaspoon chopped mint

- 1 teaspoon vegetable broth
- ¼ teaspoon salt
- ¼ teaspoon cumin
- ¼ teaspoon paprika
- ¼ teaspoon dried herbs
- ¼ teaspoon ground black pepper
- 1 tablespoon chopped fresh parsley
- 4 sliced zucchinis
- 1 small pack pasta

Directions:

In a saucepan, add green lentils, water, and broth and cook it over medium flame for around 30 minutes or until the liquid evaporates properly. Take a pan with oil and fry onion and garlic for around 2 to 3 minutes. Add tomato, remaining water, vinegar, salt, pepper, herbs, paprika, and cumin in it and cook it for around 20 minutes over low flame. In the end, add parsley and mint in it. Now add cooked lentils in it and whisk well. Cook it for few minutes. Prepare the pasta according to the given directions and serve it with the prepared sauce.

Nutrition:

Carbohydrates 56g, protein 16g, fats 1.8g, calories 295, sugar 8.4g

Lemon Pepper Asparagus Pasta

Preparation time: 10 minutes
Cooking time: 15 minutes
Servings: 4

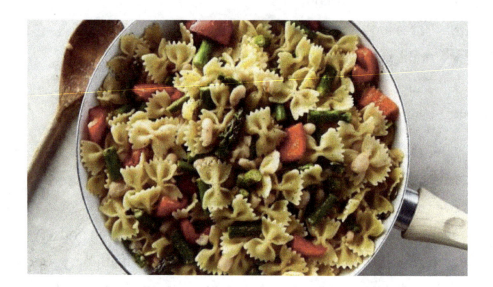

Ingredients:

- 2 lb. Sliced and trimmed asparagus
- 5 tablespoons olive oil
- 3 tablespoons lemon juice
- 8 oz. Fettuccine
- 2 tablespoons minced garlic cloves
- 1 tablespoon shredded lemon zest
- ¼ teaspoon ground black pepper
- 1 diced red bell pepper
- 1/8 teaspoon crushed red chili

- 1 tablespoon honey

Directions:

In a bowl, add lemon juice, honey, garlic, lemon zest, and olive oil. Whisk all the ingredients well. Cook pasta according to the given directions and drain well. Place a skillet over medium flame and cook asparagus for 2 minutes. Add red peppers in it and cook it for around 2 minutes more. Combine the prepared mixture in it and whisk it well. It is ready to serve.

Nutrition:

Carbohydrates 45g, protein 12g, fats 17g, calories 378

Butternut Squash Fettuccine

Preparation time: 25 minutes
Cooking time: 15 minutes
Servings: 6

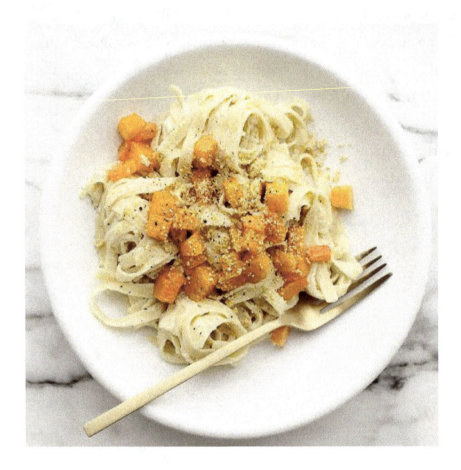

Ingredients:

- 1-pound fettuccine
- 1-pound diced butternut squash
- ¾ cup heavy cream

- 2 ounces shredded parmesan
- 3 tablespoons diced unsalted butter
- ¼ teaspoon salt
- ½ teaspoon shredded nutmeg
- ¾ cup of water

Directions:

In a pan, add butter squash, butter and water and cook it over medium flame. When it starts, boiling reduces the flame and cooks it for around 15 minutes. With the help of a blender, make the puree of the squash. Season it with salt and nutmeg. Cook the pasta according to the given directions. Place the cooked pasta and parmesan in the squash sauce, stir it well, and serve it.

Nutrition:

Carbohydrates 63g, protein 11g, fats 5.9g, calories 335, sugar 1.3g

Collard Green Spaghetti

Preparation time: 10 minutes
Cooking time: 10 minutes
Servings: 2

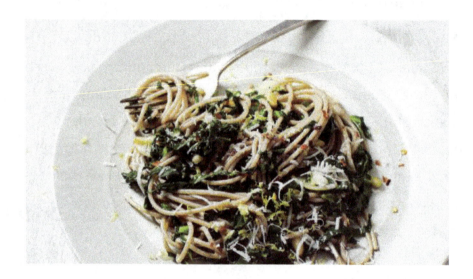

Ingredients:

- 8ounces fresh collard greens
- ½ of one pack of the whole what thing spaghetti
- Big pinch red pepper flakes
- 3 tbsp of pine nuts
- Sea salt
- Olive oil
- Black pepper
- 2 small cloves garlic
- 1-ounce parmesan cheese

- ½ of lemon [cut into wedges]

Directions:

Add salted water in a big pot and bring it to boil. Add pasta to the pot and cook it as per the directions. Drain water when it is done and keep the pasta aside. Take the collard green and cut out the center rib of each. Combine the green together and roll them in a cigar-like shape. Now slice then vertically in as thin as possible size. Chop the strands from the center to make them long.

Take a 12-inch skillet and heat it on medium heat. Now, add pine nuts to the skillet and toast it until fragrant and brown in color. Take the nuts out of the skillet and save for later. Now add one tbsp. Of olive oil in the skillet and heat it on medium. Add garlic, pepper flakes to the oil, and stir a bit. When it starts to simmer, toss all the collard greens in it. Add salt to taste in the skillet and stir them to sauté for about three minutes.

It is time to mix up everything. Now remove the pan from heat, add greens to pasta pot and toss them together. Add a bit of olive oil in the bowl. Dish out the pasta onto a plate and top it with pine nuts, parmesan shavings and lemon wedges.

Pasta Salad with Tahini Dressing

Preparation time: 10 minutes
Cooking time: 12 minutes
Servings: 6

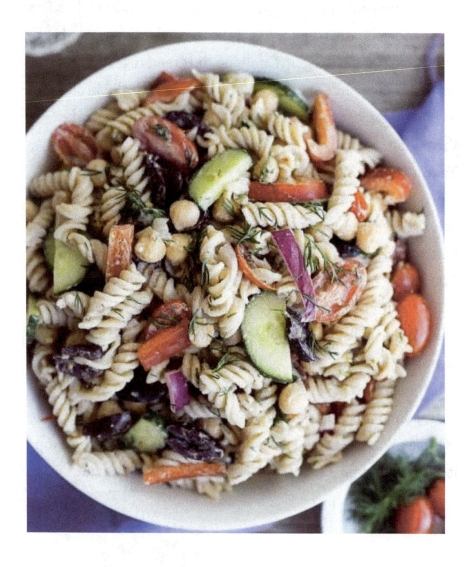

Ingredients:

- 12 ounces whole-wheat pasta
- 1 small red pepper [chopped]
- 1 ½ cup cucumber [chopped]
- 15 ounces chickpeas [drained and rinsed]
- 1 ½ cup cherry tomatoes [sliced in half]
- ½ cup red onion [sliced]
- ½ cup kalamata olives [sliced in half]
- 2 tbsp dill [chopped]
- Red pepper flakes [to taste]
- Creamy tahini sauce
- 1/3 cup tahini
- 2 cloves garlic [minced]
- Juice one lemon
- 1/3 cup of water
- ½ tsp salt

Directions:

Heat water in a large pot and cook pasta as per the packaging directions. Now add all the dressing ingredients in a large bowl and mix them well. Whisk all the sauce ingredients to make a fluffy sauce. Now add cooked pasta to the blow and toss it properly. You can serve it hot and chilled as per choice.

Nutrition:

Carbohydrates 47g, protein 20g, fats 19g, calories 349, sugar 2.5g

Spicy Vegan Pasta with Sausage

Preparation time: 5 minutes
Cooking time: 20 minutes
Servings: 6

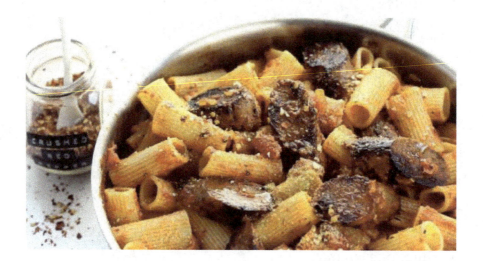

Ingredients:

- 450 grams rigatoni or pasta of choice
- 2 tbsp olive oil
- 3 vegan sausages
- ½ yellow onion [chopped]
- 3 cloves garlic [minced]
- ½ tsp red pepper flakes
- 650ml tomato paste
- Parmesan [for garnish]

Directions:

Prepare the pasta as per the package directions.

Slice the sausages in a diagonal shape with good thickness and toss them in a heated pan with a bit of olive oil on medium heat. Let each side brown evenly and remove from the pan for later use.

Put the pan back on medium heat and add one tablespoon of olive oil in it. Sauté onion and garlic in oil for about 4 minutes until online become translucent. Add pepper flakes and cook the onion for more one minute. Add tomato sauce to the pan and heat it for a while. Once it starts to simmer, add sausages and pasta to the sauce. Toss is for a little and remove the pan from the heat. Once everything is mixed, then serve is with a sprinkle of parmesan.

Nutrition:

Carbohydrates 72g, protein 28g, fats 10g, calories 482, sugar 9g

Chapter 11: Vegetables

Tahini Broccoli Slaw

Preparation time: 15 minutes
Cooking time: 0 minutes
Servings: 4 to 6 servings

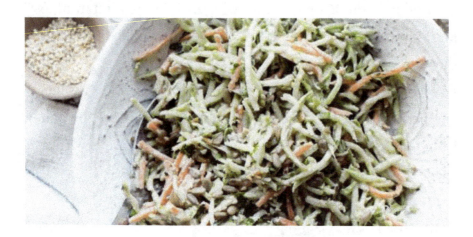

Ingredients:

- ¼ cup tahini (sesame paste)
- 2 tablespoons white miso
- 1 tablespoon rice vinegar
- 1 tablespoon toasted sesame oil
- 2 teaspoons soy sauce
- 1 (12-ounce) bag broccoli slaw
- 2 green onions, minced
- ¼ cup toasted sesame seeds

Directions:

In a large bowl, whisk together the tahini, miso, vinegar, oil, and soy sauce. Add the broccoli slaw, green onions, and sesame seeds and toss to coat.

Set aside for 20 minutes before serving.

Steamed Cauliflower

Preparation time: 5 minutes
Cooking time: 10 minutes
Servings: 6

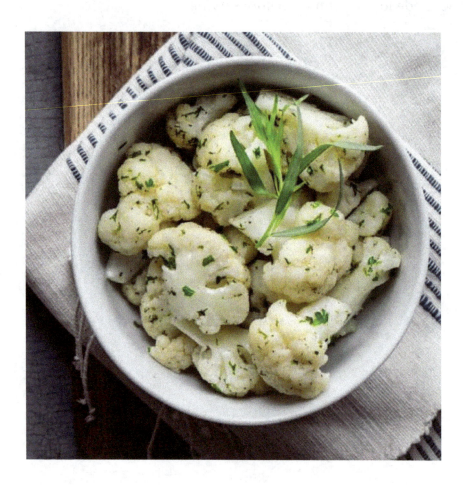

Ingredients:

- 1 large head cauliflower
- 1 cup water
- ½ teaspoon salt

- 1 teaspoon red pepper flakes (optional)

Directions:

Preparing the ingredients.

Remove any leaves from the cauliflower, and cut it into florets. In a large saucepan, bring the water to a boil. Place a steamer basket over the water, and add the florets and salt. Cover and steam for 5 to 7 minutes, until tender. In a large bowl, toss the cauliflower with the red pepper flakes (if using). Transfer the florets to a large airtight container or 6 single-serving containers. Let cool before sealing the lids.

Nutrition: calories: 35; fat: 0g; protein: 3g; carbohydrates: 7g; fiber: 4g; sugar: 4g; sodium: 236mg

Roasted Cauliflower Tacos

Preparation time: 10 minutes
Cooking time: 30 minutes
Servings: 8 tacos

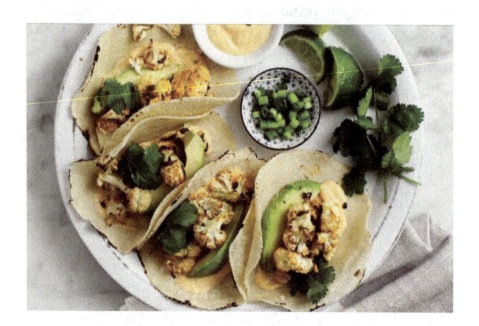

Ingredients:

For the roasted cauliflower:

- 1 head cauliflower, cut into bite-size pieces
- 1 tablespoon olive oil (optional)
- 2 tablespoons whole-wheat flour
- 2 tablespoons nutritional yeast
- 1 to 2 teaspoons smoked paprika
- ½ to 1 teaspoon chili powder
- Pinch sea salt

For the tacos:

- 2 cups shredded lettuce
- 2 cups cherry tomatoes, quartered
- 2 carrots, scrubbed or peeled, and grated
- ½ cup fresh mango salsa
- ½ cup guacamole
- 8 small whole-grain or corn tortillas
- 1 lime, cut into 8 wedges

Directions:

To make the roasted cauliflower

Preheat the oven to 350°f. Lightly grease a large rectangular baking sheet with olive oil, or line it with parchment paper. In a large bowl, toss the cauliflower pieces with oil (if using), or just rinse them so they're wet. The idea is to get the seasonings to stick. In a smaller bowl, mix together the flour, nutritional yeast, paprika, chili powder, and salt.

Add the seasonings to the cauliflower, and mix it around with your hands to thoroughly coat. Spread the cauliflower on the baking sheet, and roast for 20 to 30 minutes, or until softened.

To make the tacos

Prep the veggies, salsa, and guacamole while the cauliflower is roasting. Once the cauliflower is cooked, heat the tortillas for just a few minutes in the oven or in a small skillet. Set everything out on the table, and assemble your tacos as you go. Give a squeeze of fresh lime just before eating.

Per serving (1 taco): calories: 198; total fat: 6g; carbs: 32g; fiber: 6g; protein: 7g

Cajun Sweet Potatoes

Preparation time: 5 minutes

Cooking time: 30 minutes

es

Servings: 4

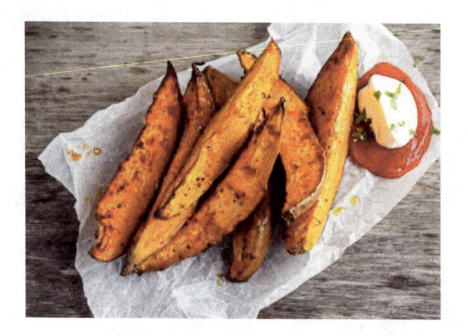

Ingredients:

- 2 pounds sweet potatoes
- 2 teaspoons extra-virgin olive oil
- ½ teaspoon ground cayenne pepper
- ½ teaspoon smoked paprika
- ½ teaspoon dried oregano
- ½ teaspoon dried thyme

- ½ teaspoon garlic powder
- ½ teaspoon salt (optional)

Directions:

Preparing the ingredients.

Preheat the oven to 400°f. Line a baking sheet with parchment paper.

Wash the potatoes, pat dry, and cut into ¾-inch cubes. Transfer to a large bowl, and pour the olive oil over the potatoes.

In a small bowl, combine the cayenne, paprika, oregano, thyme, and garlic powder. Sprinkle the spices over the potatoes and combine until the potatoes are well coated.

Spread the potatoes on the prepared baking sheet in a single layer. Season with the salt (if using). Roast for 30 minutes, stirring the potatoes after 15 minutes.

Divide the potatoes evenly among 4 single-serving containers. Let cool completely before sealing.

Nutrition: calories: 219; fat: 3g; protein: 4g; carbohydrates: 46g; fiber: 7g; sugar: 9g; sodium: 125mg

Creamy Mint-Lime Spaghetti Squash

Preparation time: 10 minutes
Cooking time: 30 minutes
Servings: 3

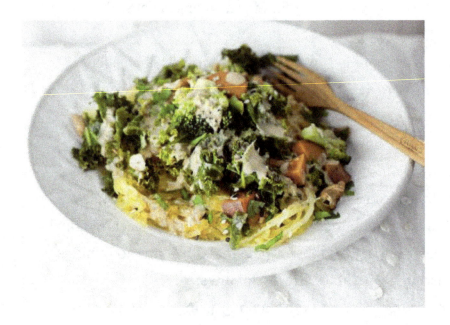

Ingredients:

For the dressing:

- 3 tablespoons tahini
- Zest and juice of 1 small lime
- 2 tablespoons fresh mint, minced
- 1 small garlic clove, pressed
- 1 tablespoon nutritional yeast
- Pinch sea salt

For the spaghetti squash:

- 1 spaghetti squash
- Pinch sea salt
- 1 cup cherry tomatoes, chopped
- 1 cup chopped bell pepper, any color
- Freshly ground black pepper

Directions:

To make the dressing

Make the dressing by whisking together the tahini and lime juice until thick, stirring in water if you need it, until smooth, then add the rest of the ingredients. Or you can purée all the ingredients in a blender.

To make spaghetti

Carefully remove the squash from the pot and let it cool until you can safely handle it. Set half the squash aside for another meal. Scoop out the squash from the skin, which stays hard like a shell, and break the strands apart. The flesh absorbs water while boiling, so set the "noodles" in a strainer for 10 minutes, tossing occasionally to drain. Transfer the cooked spaghetti squash to a large bowl and toss with the mint-lime dressing. Then top with the cherry tomatoes and bell pepper. Add an extra sprinkle of nutritional yeast and black pepper, if you wish.

Nutrition: calories: 199; total fat: 10g; carbs: 27g; fiber: 5g; protein: 7g

Smoky Coleslaw

Preparation time: 10 minutes
Cooking time: 0 minutes
Servings: 6

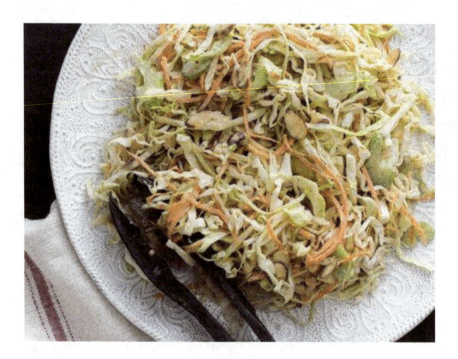

Ingredients:

- 1-pound shredded cabbage
- ⅓ cup vegan mayonnaise
- ¼ cup unseasoned rice vinegar
- 3 tablespoons plain vegan yogurt or plain soymilk
- 1 tablespoon vegan sugar
- ½ teaspoon salt
- ¼ teaspoon freshly ground black pepper

- ¼ teaspoon smoked paprika
- ¼ teaspoon chipotle powder

Directions:

Preparing the ingredients.

Put the shredded cabbage in a large bowl. In a medium bowl, whisk the mayonnaise, vinegar, yogurt, sugar, salt, pepper, paprika, and chipotle powder.

Pour over the cabbage, and mix with a spoon or spatula and until the cabbage shreds are coated. Divide the coleslaw evenly among 6 single-serving containers. Seal the lids.

Nutrition: calories: 73; fat: 4g; protein: 1g; carbohydrates: 8g; fiber: 2g; sugar: 5g; sodium: 283mg

Simple Sesame Stir-Fry

Preparation time: 10 minutes
Cooking time: 20 minutes
Servings: 4

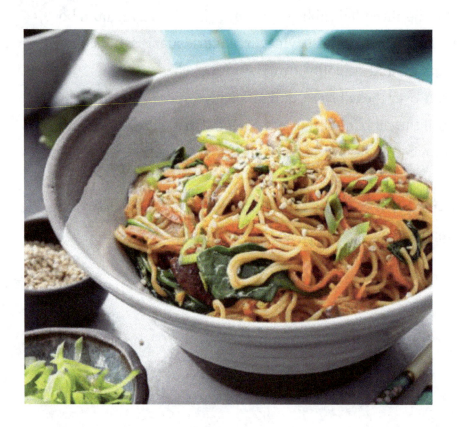

Ingredients:

- 1 cup quinoa
- 2 cups water
- Pinch sea salt
- 1 head broccoli
- 1 to 2 teaspoons untoasted sesame oil, or olive oil

- 1 cup snow peas, or snap peas, ends trimmed and cut in half
- 1 cup frozen shelled edamame beans, or peas
- 2 cups chopped swiss chard, or other large-leafed green
- 2 scallions, chopped
- 2 tablespoons water
- 1 teaspoon toasted sesame oil
- 1 tablespoon tamari, or soy sauce
- 2 tablespoons sesame seeds

Directions:

Preparing the ingredients.

Put the quinoa, water, and sea salt in a medium pot, bring it to a boil for a minute, then turn to low and simmer, covered, for 20 minutes. The quinoa is fully cooked when you see the swirl of the grains with a translucent center, and it is fluffy. Do not stir the quinoa while it is cooking.

Meanwhile, cut the broccoli into bite-size florets, cutting and pulling apart from the stem. Also chop the stem into bite-size pieces. Heat a large skillet to high, and sauté the broccoli in the untoasted sesame oil, with a pinch of salt to help it soften. Keep this moving continuously, so that it doesn't burn, and add an extra drizzle of oil if needed as you add the rest of the vegetables.

Add the snow peas next, continuing to stir. Add the edamame until they thaw.

Add the swiss chard and scallions at the same time, tossing for only a minute to wilt. Then add 2 tablespoons of water to the hot skillet so that it sizzles and finishes the vegetables with a quick steam.

Dress with the toasted sesame oil and tamari, and toss one last time. Remove from the heat immediately. Serve a scoop of cooked quinoa, topped with stir-fry and sprinkled with some sesame seeds, and an extra drizzle of tamari and/or toasted sesame oil if you like.

Nutrition: calories: 334; total fat: 13g; carbs: 42g; fiber: 9g; protein: 17g

Mediterranean Hummus Pizza

Preparation time: 10 minutes
Cooking time: 30 minutes
Servings: 2 pizzas

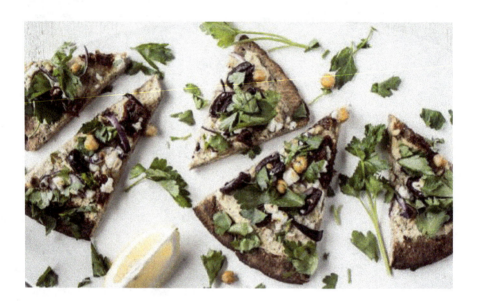

Ingredients:

- ½ zucchini, thinly sliced
- ½ red onion, thinly sliced
- 1 cup cherry tomatoes, halved
- 2 to 4 tablespoons pitted and chopped black olives
- Pinch sea salt
- Drizzle olive oil (optional)
- 2 prebaked pizza crusts
- ½ cup classic hummus, or roasted red pepper hummus

- 2 to 4 tablespoons cheesy sprinkle

Directions:

Preparing the ingredients.

Preheat the oven to 400°f. Place the zucchini, onion, cherry tomatoes, and olives in a large bowl, sprinkle them with the sea salt, and toss them a bit. Drizzle with a bit of olive oil (if using), to seal in the flavor and keep them from drying out in the oven.

Lay the two crusts out on a large baking sheet. Spread half the hummus on each crust, and top with the veggie mixture and some cheesy sprinkle. Pop the pizzas in the oven for 20 to 30 minutes, or until the veggies are soft.

Per serving (1 pizza) calories: 500; total fat: 25g; carbs: 58g; fiber: 12g; protein: 19g

Baked Brussels Sprouts

Preparation time: 10 minutes
Cooking time: 40 minutes
Servings: 4

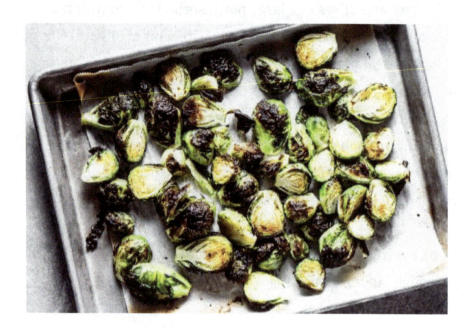

Ingredients:

- 1-pound brussels sprouts
- 2 teaspoons extra-virgin olive or canola oil
- 4 teaspoons minced garlic (about 4 cloves)
- 1 teaspoon dried oregano
- ½ teaspoon dried rosemary
- ½ teaspoon salt
- ¼ teaspoon freshly ground black pepper
- 1 tablespoon balsamic vinegar

Directions:

Preparing the ingredients.

Preheat the oven to 400°f. Line a rimmed baking sheet with parchment paper. Trim and halve the brussels sprouts. Transfer to a large bowl. Toss with the olive oil, garlic, oregano, rosemary, salt, and pepper to coat well.

Transfer to the prepared baking sheet. Bake for 35 to 40 minutes, shaking the pan occasionally to help with even browning, until crisp on the outside and tender on the inside. Remove from the oven and transfer to a large bowl. Stir in the balsamic vinegar, coating well.

Divide the brussels sprouts evenly among 4 single-serving containers. Let cool before sealing the lids.

Nutrition: calories: 77; fat: 3g; protein: 4g; carbohydrates: 12g; fiber: 5g; sugar: 3g; sodium: 320mg

Minted Peas

Preparation time: 5 minutes
Cooking time: 5 minutes
Servings: 4

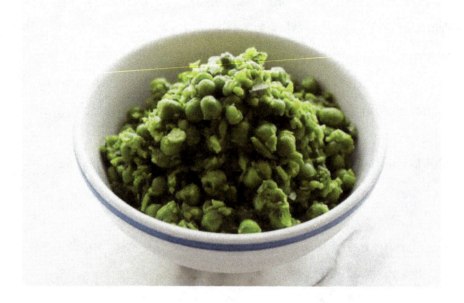

Ingredients:

- 1 tablespoon olive oil
- 4 cups peas, fresh or frozen (not canned)
- ½ teaspoon sea salt
- Freshly ground black pepper
- 3 tablespoons chopped fresh mint

Directions:

Preparing the ingredients.

In a large sauté pan, heat the olive oil over medium-high heat until hot. Add the peas and cook, about 5 minutes.

Remove the pan from heat. Stir in the salt, season with pepper, and stir in the mint.

Serve hot.

Spicy Fruit and Veggie Gazpacho

Preparation time: 10 minutes
Cooking time: 0 minutes
Servings: 8

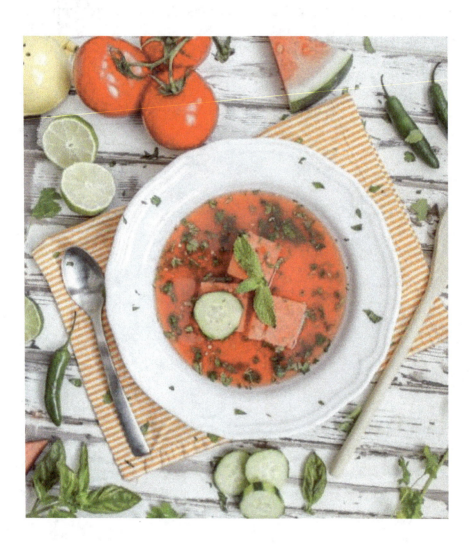

Ingredients:

- 2 large tomatoes
- 1 serrano chile, seeded
- 4 cups cubed fresh watermelon, divided
- 2 teaspoons unseasoned rice vinegar or white wine vinegar
- ¼ cup extra-virgin olive oil or 2 to 3 tablespoons vegetable broth
- 1 large cucumber, peeled, seeded, and diced
- 1 small red onion, diced
- 1 small red bell pepper, seeded and diced
- ¼ cup minced fresh dill
- Salt
- Freshly ground black pepper

Directions:

Preparing the ingredients.

In a blender, purée the tomatoes, chile, and 2 cups of watermelon. Pour in the vinegar and olive oil and pulse. Add the cucumber, onion, bell pepper, and dill and purée until smooth. Taste before seasoning with salt and black pepper.

In a large bowl, pour the gazpacho over the remaining 2 cups of watermelon. Scoop 1½ cups of gazpacho into each of 8 single-serving containers. Seal the lids.

Nutrition: calories: 106; fat: 7g; protein: 2g; carbohydrates: 12g; fiber: 2g; sugar: 8g; sodium: 28mg

Maple Dijon Burgers

Preparation time: 20 minutes
Cooking time: 30 minutes
Servings: 12 burgers

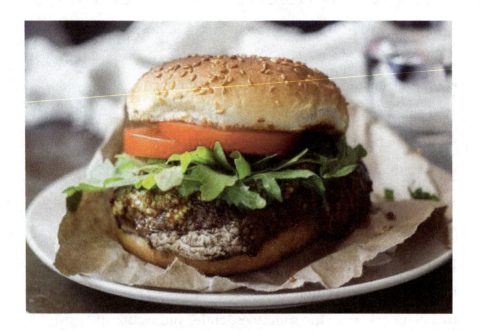

Ingredients:

- 1 red bell pepper
- 1 (19-ounce) can chickpeas, rinsed and drained, or 2 cups cooked
- 1 cup ground almonds
- 2 teaspoons Dijon mustard
- 2 teaspoons maple syrup
- 1 garlic clove, pressed

- Juice of ½ lemon
- 1 teaspoon dried oregano
- ½ teaspoon dried sage
- 1 cup spinach
- 1 to 1½ cups rolled oats

Directions:

Preparing the ingredients.

Preheat the oven to 350°f. Line a large baking sheet with parchment paper.

Cut the red pepper in half, remove the stem and seeds, and put on the baking sheet cut side up in the oven. Roast in the oven while you prep the other ingredients.

Put the chickpeas in the food processor, along with the almonds, mustard, maple syrup, garlic, lemon juice, oregano, sage, and spinach. Pulse until things are thoroughly combined but not puréed. When the red pepper is softened a bit, about 10 minutes, add it to the processor along with the oats and pulse until they are chopped just enough to form patties. If you don't have a food processor, mash the chickpeas with a potato masher or fork, and make sure everything else is chopped up as finely as possible, then stir together.

Scoop up ¼-cup portions and form into 12 patties, and lay them out on the baking sheet. Put the burgers in the oven and bake until the outside is lightly browned, about 30 minutes.

Per serving (1 burger): calories: 200; total fat: 11g; carbs: 21g; fiber: 6g; protein: 8g

Caramelized Root Vegetables

Preparation time: 5 minutes

Cooking time: 25 minutes

Servings: 4 servings

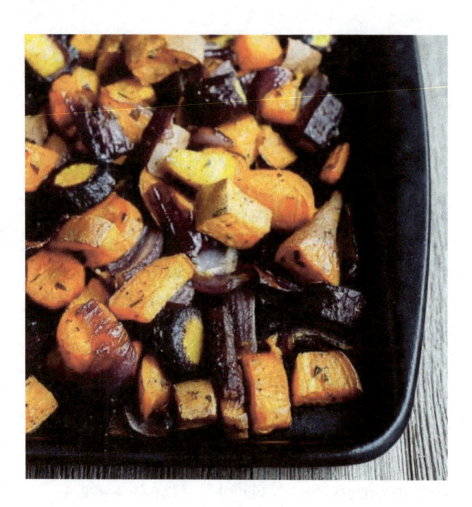

Ingredients:

- 2 tablespoons olive oil
- 2 garlic cloves, minced

- 4 medium shallots, halved or quartered
- 3 large carrots, cut into 1-inch chunks
- 3 large parsnips, cut into 1-inch chunks
- 2 small turnips, cut into 1-inch dice
- 1/2 cup light brown sugar
- 1/4 cup water
- 1/4 cup sherry vinegar
- Salt and freshly ground black pepper

Directions:

In a large skillet, heat the oil over medium heat. Add the garlic and shallots and cook for 1 minute to soften. Add the carrots, parsnips, and turnips and cook, stirring, until lightly brown and softened, about 5 minutes.

Stir in the sugar and 2 tablespoons of the water and cook, stirring until the sugar dissolves, about 5 minutes.

Stir in the remaining 2 tablespoons water and the vinegar and simmer for 2 to 3 minutes to blend the flavors. Season with salt and pepper to taste. Cover and cook on low until the vegetables are soft, about 25 minutes, stirring occasionally. Serve immediately.

Sushi-Style Quinoa

Preparation time: 2 minutes
Cooking time: 25 minutes
Servings: 4

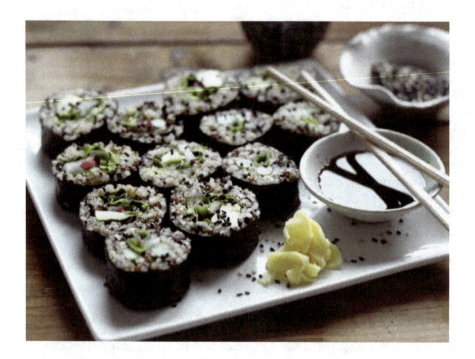

Ingredients:

- 2 cups water
- 1 cup dry quinoa, rinsed
- ¼ cup unseasoned rice vinegar
- ¼ cup mirin or white wine vinegar

Directions:

Preparing the ingredients.

In a large saucepan, bring the water to a boil. Add the quinoa to the boiling water, stir, cover, and reduce the heat to low. Simmer for 15 to 20 minutes, until the liquid is absorbed. Remove from the heat and let stand for 5 minutes.

Fluff with a fork. Add the vinegar and mirin, and stir to combine well.

Divide the quinoa evenly among 4 mason jars or single-serving containers. Let cool before sealing the lids.

Nutrition: calories: 192; fat: 3g; protein: 6g; carbohydrates: 34g; fiber: 3g; sugar: 4g; sodium: 132mg

Pepper Medley

Preparation time: 10 minutes
Cooking time: 15 minutes
Servings: 4

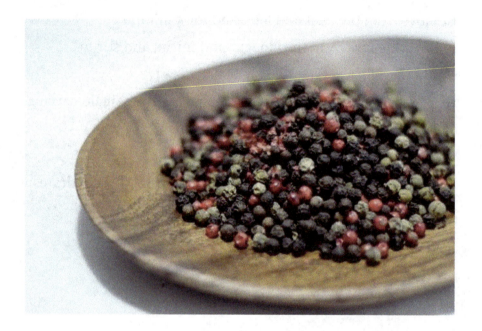

Ingredients:

- 3 tablespoons olive oil
- 1 red bell pepper, sliced
- 1 orange bell pepper, sliced
- 1 yellow bell pepper, sliced
- 1 green bell pepper, sliced
- 2 garlic cloves, minced
- 3 tablespoons red wine vinegar

- Sea salt
- Freshly ground black pepper
- 2 tablespoons chopped fresh basil

Directions:

Preparing the ingredients.

In a large sauté pan, heat the olive oil over medium-high heat until it shimmers. Add the bell peppers and cook, stirring frequently, until softened, 7 to 10 minutes. Add the garlic and cook until it is fragrant, about 30 seconds. Add the vinegar, using a spoon to scrape any browned bits off the bottom of the pan.

Simmer until the vinegar reduces, 2 to 3 minutes. Season with salt and pepper. Stir in the basil and serve immediately.

Sautéed Citrus Spinach

Preparation time: 10 minutes
Cooking time: 10 minutes
Servings: 4

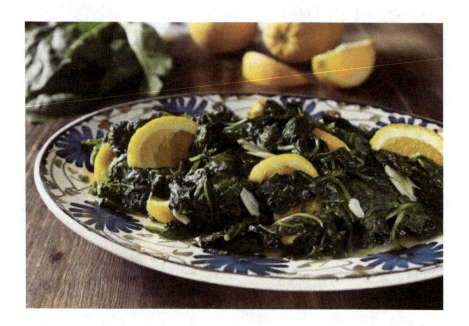

Ingredients:

- 2 tablespoons olive oil
- 1 shallot, chopped
- 2 garlic cloves, minced
- 10 ounces baby spinach
- Zest and juice of 1 orange
- Sea salt
- Freshly ground black pepper

Directions:

Preparing the ingredients.

In a large sauté pan, heat the olive oil over medium-high heat until it shimmers. Add the shallot and cook until soft, about 3 minutes. Add the garlic and cook until it is fragrant, about 30 seconds. Add the spinach, orange juice, and orange zest.

Cook, stirring, until the spinach wilts, 2 to 3 minutes. Season with salt and pepper.

Serve warm.

Chapter 12: Snacks/Desserts

Strawberry Mango Shave Ice

Preparation time: 5 hours 30 minutes
Cooking time: 0 minutes
Servings: 3

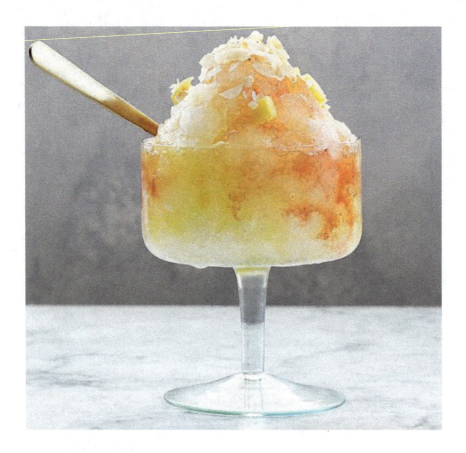

Ingredients:

- ½ cup superfine sugar, divided
- 1½ cups mango juice
- 1 diced mango
- 32 oz diced strawberries
- ½ cup coconut, toasted

Directions:

Add one cup of water and sugar to a pot over high heat and boil.

Remove from heat and add two more cups of water.

Freeze this mixture stirring once in 40 minutes.

Take a blender and add all remaining ingredients and blend until smooth.

Strain into a container with a pouring spout.

For serving, add ice into glasses and pour juice and mixture over them.

Serve and enjoy.

Nutritional value nutrition:

Calories 366

Fat 5.5 g

Carbohydrates 82.4 g

Protein 2.7 g

Chocolate Avocado Mousse

Preparation time: 10 minutes
Cooking time: 10 minutes
Servings: 6

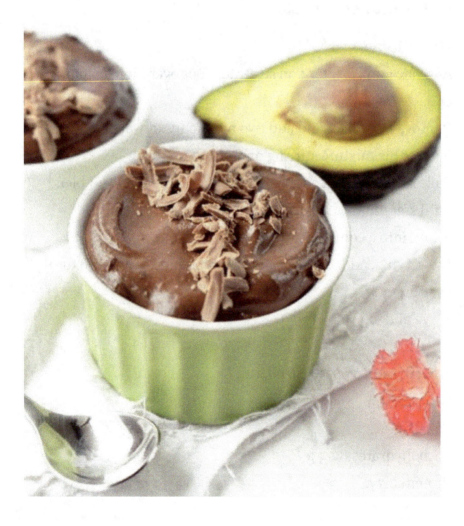

Ingredients:

- 1¼ cups almond milk, unsweetened
- 1 lb. Dark chocolate, chopped
- 4 ripe avocados, peeled and chopped
- ¼ cup syrup of agave
- 1 tbsp orange zest, finely grated
- 2 tbsp puffed quinoa
- 2 tsp sea salt
- 2 tsp pepper flakes
- 1 tbsp olive oil

Directions:

Heat almond milk in a saucepan. After 5 to 10 minutes, add in chopped chocolate.

Take all remaining ingredients and blend them till they become smooth.

Mix both and let cool for a while.

Refrigerate for about 2 hours before serving.

Nutrition:

Calories 540

Fat 43.5 g

Carbohydrates 61.2 g

Protein 6.1 g

Fudge

Preparation time: 10 minutes
Cooking time: 5 minutes
Servings: 18

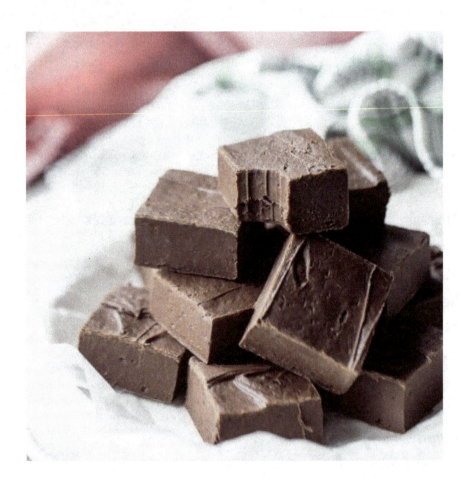

Ingredients:

- 1 cup vegan chocolate chips
- ½ cup soy milk

Directions:

Line an 8-inch portion skillet with wax paper. Set aside. Clear some space in your refrigerator for this dish as you will need it later.

Melt chocolate chips in a double boiler or add chocolate and almond spread to a medium, microwave-safe bowl. Melt it in the microwave in 20-second increments until chocolate melts. In between each 20-second burst, stir the chocolate until it is smooth.

Empty the melted chocolate mixture into the lined skillet. Tap the sides of the skillet to make sure the mixture spreads into an even layer. Alternatively, use a spoon to make swirls on top. Move skillet to the refrigerator until it is firm. Remove the skillet from the refrigerator and cut fudge into 18 squares.

Nutrition:

Calories 21

Fats 1.2 g

Carbohydrates 2.2 g

Protein 0.2 g

Chocolate Chip Cookies

Preparation time: 20 minutes
Cooking time: 0 minutes
Servings: 20

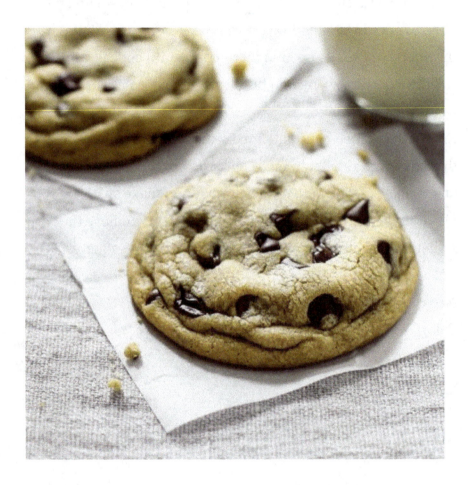

Ingredients:

- 1½ cups roasted, salted cashews
- 8 oz pitted medjool dates
- 3 tbsp coconut oil

- 2 tsp vanilla extract
- 2 cups old-fashioned oats
- 1 cup semi-sweet or dark chocolate chips

Directions:

Line a baking sheet with parchment paper.

In the bowl of a food processor, add the cashews, dates, coconut oil, vanilla, and oats.

Pulse until combined, and all lumps are broken up.

On the off chance that the batter appears to be dry, add 1 more tbsp of coconut oil and a sprinkle of water. Mix in the chocolate chips.

Divide the mixture into 18 to 20 tbsp-size balls and place them on the prepared baking sheet. Using the palm of your hand, delicately press down each ball into flat circles. Move the sheet to the refrigerator for 10 to 15 minutes or until cookies are firm.

Serve and enjoy.

Nutrition:

Calories 207

Fat 9.4 g

Carbohydrates 28.1 g

Protein 4.2 g

Pumpkin Ice Cream

Preparation time: 15 minutes
Servings: 6

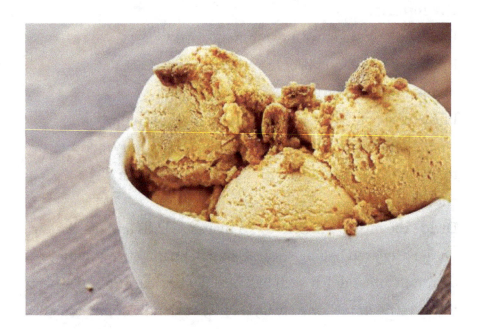

Ingredients:

- 1 can coconut milk
- 1 cup unsweetened almond milk
- 1 cup canned or fresh pumpkin puree
- 1 teaspoon pure vanilla extract
- ½ teaspoon nutmeg
- 2 ½ teaspoons ground cinnamon
- ½ teaspoon ground ginger
- Pinch of salt

- 1 tablespoon gelatin

Directions:

Dissolve the gelatin in ¼ cup boiling water.

Add the rest of the ingredients, including the gelatin mixture, to a food processor. Blend until smooth.

Transfer the mixture to a freezer-safe container. Cover. Freeze for 2 hours.

After 2 hours, use a wooden spoon to break up the ice cream in order to prevent crystalizing.

Leave in the freezer overnight. Serve the following day.

Nutritional values:

Carbohydrates: 4.5 grams
Fat: 11.3 grams
Protein: 1.3 grams

Sautéed Pears

Servings: 6

Time: 35 minutes

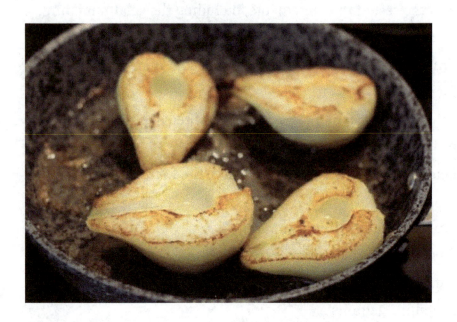

Ingredients:

- 2 tablespoons margarine (or vegan butter)
- ¼ teaspoon cinnamon
- ¼ teaspoon nutmeg
- 6 bosc pears, peeled & quartered
- 1 tablespoon lemon juice
- ½ cup walnuts, toasted & chopped (optional)

Directions:

Melt your vegan butter in a skillet, and then add your spices. Cook for a half a minute before adding in your pears.

Cook for fifteen minutes, and then stir in your lemon juice. Serve with walnuts if desired.

Nutrition:
Calories: 220
Protein: 2 grams
Fat: 10 grams
Carbs: 31 grams

Raw Vegan Chocolate Fruit Balls

Total preparation & cooking time: 5 min
Servings: 20 balls

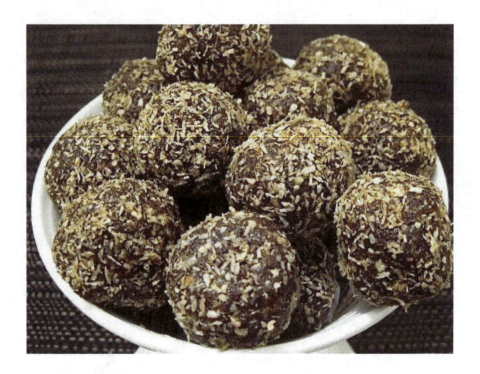

Ingredients:

- ½ cup raisins
- 1 cup nuts raw cashews, almonds, macadamias
- 2 tbsp. Cocoa powder, unsweetened
- ½ cup apricot, dried & chopped
- 1 tbsp. Orange juice, fresh
- ½ cup organic dates, pitted & chopped
- 2 drops of natural almond essence

- 1/4 cup coconut, desiccated
- 1/2 tsp. Cinnamon

Directions:

In a small bowl, mix the cinnamon and coconut together and keep it aside for rolling.

In a food processor, put all of the other ingredients, and if it doesn't get combined together completely, add in the orange juice slowly.

Make small balls from the mixture & coat the balls with coconut mixture.

Store in a refrigerator in an airtight glass container.

Nutritional value (amount per serving): 104 calories, 5.8 g total fat, 0 mg cholesterol, 12.7 g total carbohydrate, 2.3 g dietary fiber, 2.8 g protein

Baked Sesame Fries

Preparation time: 10 minutes
Cooking time: 20 minutes
Servings: 4

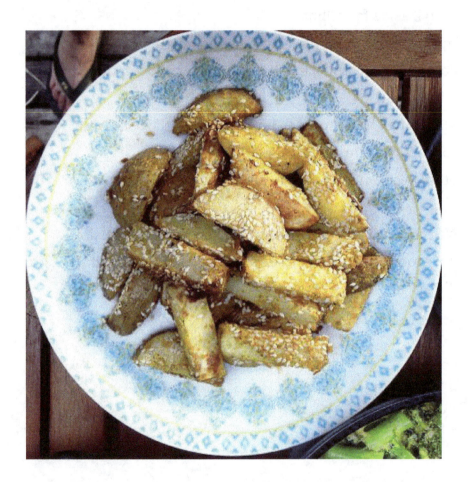

Ingredients:

- 1 lb. Yukon potatoes, gold, cut into wedges, unpeeled
- 1 tbsp avocado, grapeseed
- 2 tbsp, seeds, sesame

- 1 tbsp potato starch
- 1 tbsp, yeast nutritional
- Generous pinch salt
- Black pepper

Directions:

Preheat stove to 425°f.

Delicately oil a baking sheet of metal or line it with parchment paper.

Toss potatoes with all of the ingredients until covered, if seeds don't stick, drizzle a little more oil.

Spread potatoes in an even layer onto the prepared sheet and bake for 20 to 25 minutes, tossing once halfway through, until the potatoes become crispy.

Serve with desired toppings.

Nutrition:

Calories 192

Fat 5.9 g

Carbohydrates 32.6 g

Protein 2.8 g

No-Bake Coconut Chia Macaroons

Preparation time: 2 hours
Cooking time: 0 minutes
Servings: 6

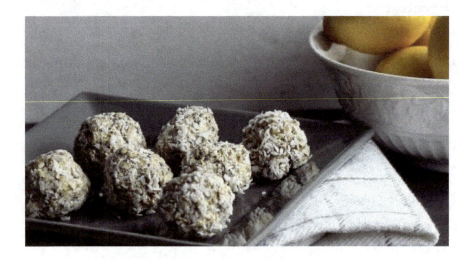

Ingredients:

- 1 cup shredded coconut
- 2 tbsp chia seeds
- ½ cup coconut cream
- ½ cup erythritol

Directions:

Combine all ingredients in a bowl. Mix until well combined.
Chill the mixture for about half an hour.
Once set, scoop the mixture into serving portions and roll into balls.
Return to the chiller for another hour.

Nutrition:

Calories 129

Carbohydrates 5 g

Fats 12 g

Protein 2 g

Avocado Lassi

Preparation time: 5 minutes
Servings: 3

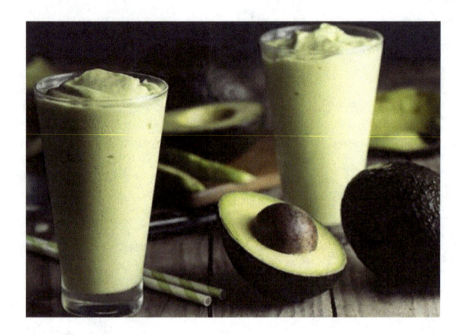

Ingredients:

- 1 avocado
- 1 cup coconut milk
- 2 cups ice cubes
- 2 tbsp erythritol
- ½ tsp powdered cardamom
- 1 tbsp vanilla extract

Directions:

Combine all ingredients in a bowl. Mix until well combined. Press the mixture into a rectangular silicone mold and freeze for an hour to set.

Slice for serving.

Nutrition:

Calories 305

Carbohydrates 9 g

Fats 29 g

Protein 3 g

Vegan Fudge Revel Bars

Preparation time: 1 hour
Servings: 12

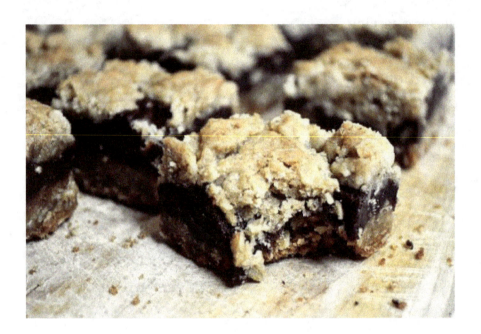

Ingredients:
- 1 cup almond flour
- ¾ cup erythritol
- ¾ cup peanut butter
- 1 tbsp vanilla extract
- ½ cup sugar-free chocolate chips
- 2 tbsp margarine

Directions:

Mix together almond butter, coconut flour, erythritol, and vanilla extract in a bowl until well combined.

Press the mixture into a rectangular silicone mold and freeze for an hour to set.

Melt the chocolate chips with the margarine for 1-2 minutes in the microwave.

Pour melted chocolate on top of the mold and chill for another hour to set.

Slice for serving.

Nutrition:

Calories 160

Carbohydrates 5 g

Fats 14 g

Protein 5 g

Chapter 13: Energizing Drinks

Gingerbread Latte

Cooking time: 10 minutes
Servings: 2

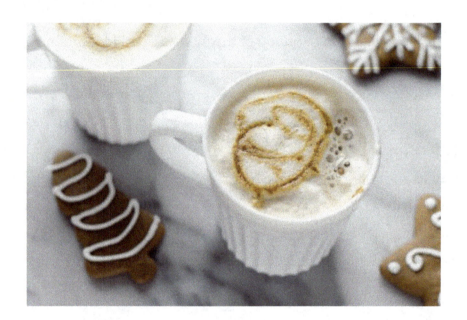

Ingredients:

- 1 tablespoon ginger, minced
- 1/2 cup espresso coffee
- 1 tablespoon sugar
- 1/2 teaspoon gingerbread spice
- 1 ½ cups coconut milk, frothed
- Whipped coconut cream

Directions:

Add ginger to a saucepan along with coffee, sugar and gingerbread spice, and bring to a boil over medium heat, and then simmer for at least 2 minutes.

When done, mix the add milk to the saucepan. Heat the mixture but do not bring to a boil.

Strain the drink and pour into the cups, and then add the coconut cream and sprinkle with the gingerbread spice. Enjoy!

Nutrition:

Calories 234

Carbohydrates 9 g

Fats 5 g

Protein 3 g

Black Forest Shake

Cooking time: 15 minutes

Servings: 2

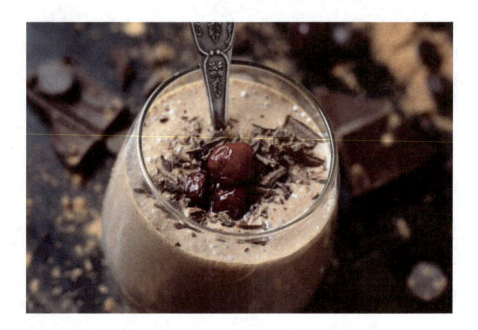

Ingredients:

For cherry compote:

- 1 tablespoon sugar
- 2 tablespoons water
- Salt, to taste
- 1 cup cherries
- 2 teaspoons lime juice

For vanilla layer:

- 1 tablespoon sugar or sweetener

- 1/2 cup coconut milk ice cubes
- Vanilla extract, to taste
- 1/2 cup vanilla ice cream

For chocolate layer:
- 1/2 cup vegan chocolate ice cream
- 2 tablespoons cherry compote
- 1/2 cup coconut milk or almond milk ice cubes
- 1 tablespoon cocoa powder
- 1 tablespoon sugar or sweetener

Directions:

Prepare cherry compote. Add all the compote ingredients to the skillet placed over medium heat, and cook until the liquid has slightly thickened and the cherries have softened. When done, let cool.

Add all the vanilla shake ingredients to a blender and process until smooth. Adjust the sweetness if needed and then scoop the mixture into the serving glasses.

Add the chocolate layer ingredients to the same blender along with 2 tablespoons of cherry compote, and then process until smooth.

Reserve some cherries for serving, and then spoon the cherry compote on top of the vanilla layer, and scoop the chocolate layer on top. Top with the reserved cherries and serve. Enjoy!

Nutrition:

Calories 125; Carbohydrates 7 g; Fats 9 g; Protein 3 g

Lemon Ginger Detox Tea

Cooking time: 5 MINUTES
Servings: 2

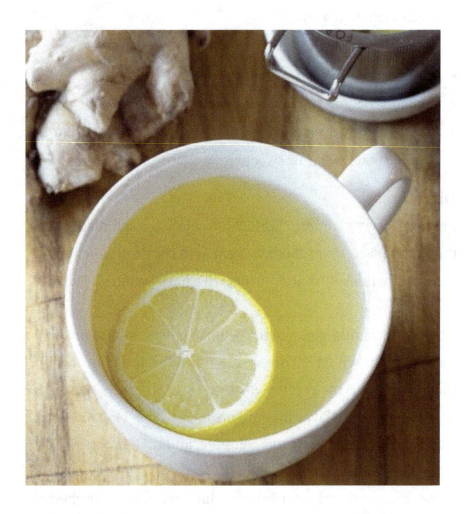

Ingredients:

- 1/2 large lemon, squeezed
- 1 ¾ cups water
- 1 small ginger knob, peeled, sliced

- Cayenne, to taste
- 1/4 teaspoon sweetener

Directions:

Boil water and then pour it into a cup. Add ginger and let rest for a few minutes and then add cayenne along with the lemon juice and sweetener.

Stir the mixture well and serve.

Enjoy!

Nutrition:

Calories 300

Carbohydrates 9 g

Fats 9 g

Protein 3 g

Carrot Pineapple Ginger Juice

Cooking time: 5 minutes

Servings: 2

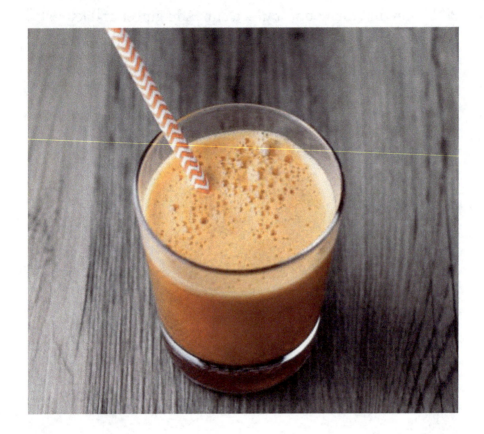

Ingredients:

- 1 small ginger knob
- 1/4 pineapple, fresh
- 9 carrots

Directions:

Add all the ingredients to a juicer and juice well.

Stir well to combine. Pour into chilled glasses and serve.

Nutrition:

Calories 305

Carbohydrates 9 g

Fats 8 g

Protein 4 g

Strawberry Shrub Mocktail

Cooking time: 5 minutes
Servings: 2

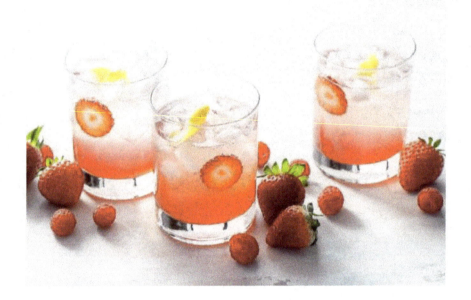

Ingredients:

- ¾ oz. Strawberry shrub
- 2 fresh basil leaves
- 2 strawberries
- 1 strip lemon zest
- 5 oz. Plain seltzer, cold
- 3 ice cubes

Directions:

Add basil leaves to a jar along with lemon zest and strawberries, and then mash well until fragrant.

Add the ice and strawberry shrub into the jar mixture and then close the lid. Shake the mixture well for 30 seconds until cold and then strain the mixture into the champagne flute.

When done, top with seltzer and enjoy!

Nutrition:

Calories 305

Carbohydrates 9 g

Fats 29 g

Protein 3 g

Strawberry Margaritas

Cooking time: 10 minutes

Servings: 2

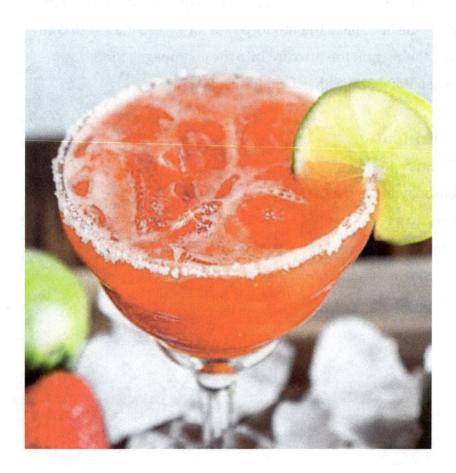

Ingredients:

- ½ cup water
- ⅛ teaspoon salt
- ¼ cup lime juice

Directions:

Add all the ingredients except lime slices to a blender. Blitz until combined and smooth.

Pour into chilled glasses and garnish with the lime slices.

Nutrition:

Calories 215

Carbohydrates 7 g

Fats 5 g

Protein 3 g

Fresh Mint Julep

Cooking time: 15 minutes
Servings: 2

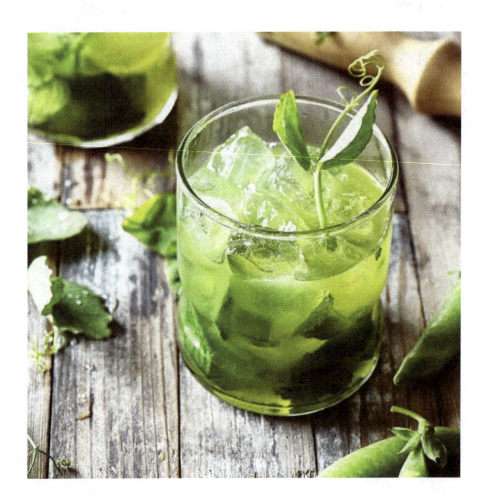

Ingredients:

- 1 cup water
- ½ cup sugar
- ½ cup sugar snap peas, trimmed, halved

- 1 cup fresh mint leaves
- 1 ½ cups bourbon
- 1 cup pea greens, chopped
- 8 cups ice cubes
- ⅓ cup lemon juice
- Salt, to taste
- Pea blossoms, for garnish

Directions:

Add sugar along with a half cup of water to a saucepan and then bring to a boil. Turn the heat off and stir in the pea greens, and then let rest for about 25 minutes. Then strain the syrup into a bowl and refrigerate for about 30 minutes until cold.

Pour the remaining cup of water into a blender along with snap peas and blend for a minute, and then pour into a bowl through a sieve. Refrigerate for about 30 minutes until cold. Prepare the cocktails. Add 2 tablespoons of mint to a glass along with 1 ½ tablespoons of the prepared syrup, and then mash the mint. When done, pour 2 teaspoons of lemon juice to the glass along with a tablespoon of pea juice and 3 tablespoons of the bourbon, and then add a half cup of the ice cubes and stir well. Garnish with mint, pea blossoms and extra pea greens.

Nutrition:

Calories 305; Carbohydrates 9 g; Fats 29 g; Protein 3 g

Conclusion

Having the right information is key if you want to make the most informed decisions in your life. Unfortunately, in the health and diet industry there is plenty of misleading information, and it can be confusing and frustrating. Don't go for the quick fix. Stick to the most sustainable, logical, healthy habits. It is said that it takes somewhere between 3 weeks and one month to create a habit. So, stick with it, and I am sure you will experience so many health benefits; you will be amazed at what you can accomplish. It is my deepest hopes that this book has been helpful to you. I hope that I have helped to bring you closer to the health you want to gain for yourself.